Mariko,
May Beauty Surround you & the Light of Spirit flow through you for yourself and all those you touch
Dancing Crow

Practical Wisdom in Natural Healing

By Deborah Frances R.N., N.D.

Polychrest Publishing
Chandler, Arizona

Practical Wisdom
in Natural Healing

Published by
Polychrest Publishing
4035 W. Chandler Blvd. #1
Chandler, AZ 85226

Cover and book design by Kalen Garr, ND
Cover photo courtesy of Tammi Miller

Printed in the United States of America

ISBN 978-0-9652376-8-0

To order addtional copies of this book, please
email: deborah.frances@yahoo.com

Dedication

THIS LITTLE BOOK IS HUMBLY DEDICATED to Mother Earth, and the plants, animals, and elementals who have so blessed my life, and to my wonderful daughter and grandson Caitlin and Connor.

In Gratitude

I FIRST WANT TO THANK MY PROOF READERS Joyce Ward and Dr. Melissa Wenzel N.D. as well as my most excellent graphic designer Dr. Kalen Garr N.D. Thanks go too to Dr. Sharol Tilgner, N.D., author of Herbal Medicine from the Heart of the Earth for all her support and persistent encouragement. Thanks to my dear friend and colleague Dr. Valeria Breiten N.D. and her dad Billy Cheek, for starting the layout process and urging me along in the writing process.

Thanks also go to my many teachers with special mention to Dr. John Collins N.D. who first introduced me to naturopathic medicine, Cascade Anderson Geller who was my first teacher of plant medicines, Dr. Rita Bettenberg N.D. whose wonderful fire matched mine and who believed in me so fully, and Annie Kahn, the Navajo Medicine Woman who insisted I stand in my power as a spiritual woman and teacher.

Finally thanks to all the many students who have appreciated my teachings. You all have been the Light of my life. Bless you and Carry On!

A Note From the Author

THIS BOOK WAS BORN OF A DESIRE TO SHARE a little of what I have learned through years of practice, and is not meant to be all inclusive. I have provided discussions and treatments, not as an attempt to offer a complete picture or treatment plan, but rather to present a few clinical pearls that have proven useful when combined with a holistic approach.

There are frequent references to the Eclectics, Eclectic prescribers, or Eclectic physicians throughout the text. This group of highly successful herbalist physicians was prominent in the late 1800s through the early 1900s. Fortunately for us, they left a legacy of writings describing very specific indications for uses of the plants they employed for medicine. Felter's book, The Eclectic Materia Medica, Pharmacology and Therapeutics, has been one of my particular favorites.

I also frequently reference the works of Dr. John Bastyr D.C., N.D. (1912 - 1995) and Dr. William "Bill" Mitchell N.D. (1947 - 2007). Both these physicians were extraordinary healers, herbalists, naturopaths, teachers and human beings.

-Deborah Frances, R.N. , N.D.

Table of Contents

Table of Contents

Chapter 1

Primary Principles of Healing

"In our study of the cause and character of disease we must endeavor to begin at the beginning, and that is LIFE itself; for the process of health, disease and cure are manifestations of that which we call life, vitality, life elements. While endeavoring to fathom the mystery of life we soon realize that we are dealing with an ultimate which no human mind is capable of solving or explaining."

-Lindlahr, Henry M.D., Philosophy of Natural Therapeutics, Maidstone Osteopathic Clinic, Maidstone, Kent, 1975

"Talker asked Annie to summarize illness, then healing. The medicine woman clapped her hands and knees together in one grand gesture. 'What causes sickness? Anything that interferes with living! Being in balance creates healing.'"

-Perrone, Stockel, & Krueger, Medicine Women, Curanderas, and Women Doctors, University of Oklahoma Press, 1989, p. 43. From an interview with Annie Kahn, Navajo Medicine Woman

Vis Medicatrix Naturae

NATUROPATHIC PHILOSOPHY, the writings of our forebears, and the results we see in clinical practice, confirm the presence of an immeasurable force that flows through the human body, and through the living medicines that are gifted to us from Nature. This immeasurable quality, Qi, vitality, vital force, energy, spiritual essence, or as Dylan Thomas so aptly put it, "the force that through the green fuse drives the flower," is the source of all healing.

Symptoms occur when the body's inherent self healing vitality responds to a potential problem, such as an injury, stress, or toxin. This natural response of the organism to a potential threat is an attempt to initiate healing, often by bringing blood and immune cells to the affected area, or by creating a discharge to eliminate toxins.

Whenever we, as patients or practitioners, interfere with this natural process, an obstacle is placed in the path to healing. Depending on the type of intervention, that obstacle can range from a simple annoyance that delays healing for a day or two, to a major wall that blocks and suppresses the organism's ability to move forward in a productive, regenerative way.

Our job as naturopaths, herbalists, and healers is to remove obstacles by choosing modalities that nourish the patient and the affected organ(s) and enhance compromised function. We may also choose to use tools that directly stimulate the innate healing mechanisms in order to hasten the healing process or to create movement where stagnation or lowered vitality threaten to block or delay complete healing.

When we follow these basic principles, symptoms will begin to subside. Sometimes this happens more rapidly than is seen in conventional medicine - not because they are suppressed, but because they are no longer necessary.

Observe the Directions of Healing

Dr. Constantine Herring, a nineteenth century homeopathic physician, made the observation that healing occurs in three directions. This law of cure or direction of healing is illustrated by the disappearance of symptoms going from within outward, from above downward, and in the reverse order from which they first appeared.

Understanding how healing flows and the directions it takes can aid the healer in discerning whether the disappearance of symptoms is in fact due to a healing response or suppression. For example, a mother brings a one year old child to the clinic with acute abundant coryza (nasal mucous discharge) and a loose cough. The child wakes frequently at night due to nasal congestion and an occasional spasmodic cough. There is a low grade fever of 99.6 (axillary) which the mother very wisely leaves alone. The physician takes the case, prescribes, and sends the mother home with instructions to follow up by phone the following day.

The next day the mother reports over the phone that her son is "so much better" and thanks the physician profusely. On further questioning, however, the prescriber discovers that the cough is no better, the child's sleep and energy have not improved, and that only the coryza has gotten better.

Herring's first Law of Cure informs us that this patient is not healing. Although the coryza has lessened, the healing is not happening from within outward. This first law informs us that the lungs, a deeper more vital organ system than the nose, should clear first, next progressing outward to the less vital organ, the nasal passages. In addition, the lack of improvement in sleep and general energy suggest that the patient's vitality has not been mobilized effectively.

Skin symptoms often give us the clearest picture of healing from above downward. A friend who had impetigo in her axillary area noted that within a few hours after taking her prescribed homeopathic remedy the eruption began to clear under her arms, but appeared lightly and transiently, first along both sides of her trunk, down the sides of her legs, and then to the top of her feet before disappearing altogether.

It has been observed that the use of the herb feverfew in treating and preventing migraine and congestive headaches sometimes results in the appearance of menstrual cramps as the headaches resolve. One herbalist stopped using the herb, because she felt the cramps were being caused by the herb, when in fact one and possibly two laws of cure are at work in these cases. The direction of above downward is clear. Once the headaches are gone and the uterine symptoms have shown themselves, the healer must follow the flow of nature and change the treatment plan to address and support this layer of healing, in this case the pelvic organs. If the patient is still benefitting from the use of the feverfew that herb should not be stopped, but continued as long as is indicated by the presence of her headaches.

The second law of cure may not be as obvious, unless the practitioner is aware that there is an increased incidence of migraine headaches in women who have suffered sexual abuse. (This does not translate to mean that all migraine sufferers have been sexually abused.) Thus we see that the feverfew is not only bringing things from above downward in a healing direction, but also operating in reverse order from which the symptoms appeared, grounding the patient's energy and bringing attention back to the area of original woundedness.

Tolle Totem: Treat the Whole Person

The physical pathologies that afflict our patients are only one aspect of the whole patient picture. Disease symptoms, although they require our attention, will be more apt to quiet down and cure when we treat the whole person. Body, mind, spirit, and emotion make up the four aspects of the patient that sits before us asking for healing. No one with a diagnosis of diabetes mellitus is going to leave the office without a dietary strategy, nutritional supplements, and herbs to help regulate their blood sugar. However, we do our patients a grave disservice if we do not remember to see the person who suffers with the diagnoses they bring into our offices.

Strong feelings can often be frightening to those of us brought up in a culture that judges and suppresses emotional expression, but the suffering that many of our patients experience often engenders powerful feelings. Those practitioners who have journeyed to the depths of their own souls with compassion and open hearted listening skills will be more able to hold a space for their patients' emotional and spiritual journeys.

Like physical symptoms, emotional and spiritual experiences must be supported, nourished, toned, and allowed to discharge without being suppressed by well-meaning advice or spiritual platitudes. Recognizing that predominant cultural views demand us to control rather than flow with the path of our soul's longing for wholeness helps us to identify and address a culturally ingrained obstacle to cure. Recognition of the obstacle is the first step to empowering its eventual removal.

Emotions considered "negative" such as anger, irritability, and resentment must be respected and honored. Although it is vital that both practitioners and patients take care not to inflict strong opinions and feelings onto others, difficult emotions do need to be heard. Making a space for patients to bring love and acceptance to the emotional body by internal dialogue or journaling with an open heart can reveal volumes about the soul's longing.

Many years ago another physician told me about a patient he was treating who had been sexually abused as a child and was struggling with anger at her mother for not protecting her.

"She has been carrying this rage for six months!" he said to me. "Can you believe it? I told her she needed to get over her anger and forgive her mother because she was just building bad karma for herself!"

This doctor's rigid spiritual beliefs and arrogant sense of superiority caused him to suppress his patient's emotional discharge by judging her process and deciding it should be different. Certainly we do not want to see our patients get stuck in any emotional process, including anger, but we have many tools to aid us in bringing movement and ultimate resolution to the patient's emotional pain without suppression and harsh judgment of their process. Simply listening and holding a sincerely compassionate, open hearted space for the patient's emotional process will often be enormously healing, as it allows the patient to feel validated, understood, and appreciated. Such active listening also offers the patient an opportunity to discharge emotions that could become toxic if held inside, thereby freeing the person to move through the emotion to the wisdom and healing that lie beneath the surface. Paradoxically, the way to transcend painful emotions is often to embrace and experience the very anguish we so wish to avoid. This approach is well described in an aphorism that remains from the writings of ancient alchemy.

"A tree's branches cannot reach to heaven until its roots have reached to hell."

While it is certainly vital that the practitioner not impede the flow of an emotional discharge, that does not necessarily mean we can allow patients to take up their entire office time emoting. Boundaries must be set that benefit both healer and patient, and as naturopathic practitioners, we have many tools to ease the way and tone the symptoms without obstructing the healing process. Flower essences, homeopathic remedies, herbal medicines, and acupuncture are a few of the tools that might be more appropriate than suppressing the patient's emotional process with a judgment or a drug.

As a registered nurse I had the opportunity to work on an acute care in-patient psychiatric ward in the local county hospital in Buffalo, New York. The skills I gained during this experience combined with my personal studies of the writings of Carl Jung, have served me throughout my career in medicine. Later, as a naturopath, I practiced for a time in an area where there was a high incidence of domestic violence. I often worked with patients who acted out the role of the abuser in their families. While many of these abusers were unable to allow themselves to be vulnerable enough to ask for help, others were more courageous. I recall one young man in his early thirties, who cried in the office as he confessed to rages that seemed to come out of nowhere and take over his whole being. His self esteem was seriously affected as he saw himself becoming the abusive father he had grown up to hate.

After letting him share his story fully, I spoke to him of the archetype of the Sacred Warrior and the need for men to heal and reclaim that aspect of masculinity.

"What you need to do is bring love and compassion to your rages," I suggested. "The judgment only makes them worse."

"What!?" he exclaimed in shock at the idea. "How can I love this terrible rage?! I lash out at my family, the ones I love the most. I am becoming just like my father!"

In this case, the patient was attempting to suppress his symptoms because he lacked the tools and guidance to integrate his inner warrior in a more constructive way. Because I had learned to be comfortable and open-hearted with my own anger, I was able to teach him and other patients like him to listen to the pain of their outraged souls with love and compassion while toning their behavior. My ability to offer him compassion stemmed from my willingness to face and integrate my own inner warrior. His naturopathic treatment plan included herbs to nourish and support his liver, adrenals, and nervous system, flower essences for easing emotional pain, and homeopathic Anacardium to help address the wounds inflicted by his personal history of abuse, all of which were vital and curative in this man's journey to wholeness.

Tolle totem includes and yet goes beyond recognition of the totality of each individual. Despite cultural conditioning that would have us believe independence is next to godliness, we are not meant to live isolated lives on islands of individual experience. Each person comes from a family, which is part of a community, a nation, a planet, and a universe, and how we live our lives affects this larger community. Each moment of life contains the memories and experiences of seven generations of our ancestors and the possibilities for seven generations of the future. Yet in our fiercely independent, individualistic culture we believe that what happens in our lives is personal to us, perhaps even caused by us, while in fact we are all influenced by the wounds and gifts of our ancestors and the generations who will come after us, living out a collective human adventure that we experience in a personal way. The pain and the joy that we feel along the journey are all part of the process of being human. Each wound that we carry is a piece of collective consciousness, an aspect of the human condition, which we have picked up to heal, not just for ourselves, but for all of humanity including past, present, and future generations.

It is important that we stop judging ourselves for being in pain or being "imperfect." We are, each of us, just as we are meant to be. Our task is to love ourselves fully, as we are, in even our most pitiful moments. It is only then that our souls can unfold to transform into who we are meant to become. It is only then that we will be able to offer the wisdom and compassion our patients so desperately seek.

Tolle Causum: Treat the Cause

"The primary cause of disease, barring accidental or surgical injury to the human organism and surroundings hostile to human life, is violation of Nature's Laws."

-Lindlahr, Henry M.D., Nature Cure: Philosophy and Practice Based on the Unity of Disease and Cure, Wildside Press, Holicong, PA, 1922, p. 21

From a naturopathic point of view, disease occurs when an individual or culture no longer lives in balance with nature. Transgression of the laws of nature results in lowered vitality and toxemia which then produce suboptimal function of organs and disease. The laws of nature are immutable. As much as we might like to believe otherwise, these laws cannot be manipulated to suit our fancies. When we choose to separate ourselves from nature in the delusion that we can successfully dominate and dishonor her laws, we eventually reap the consequences of our actions.

Honoring the ways of Mother Nature includes walking in balance with the rest of Creation. We must abandon the ludicrous assumption, so ingrained in the modern mind, that we are in some manner superior to the other species on our planet and return to the practice of honoring the plants and animals who feed us, recognizing that all living beings deserve to be treated with only the utmost respect.

How healing can a medicine be when it relies on laboratory experiments performed on animals, especially if we acknowledge that our primary wound, as a culture, is a separation from nature? How limited are we in our use of botanical medicine if we insist on viewing medicinal plants as no more than a collection of biochemical constituents, rather than living beings whose wisdom and compassion so often surpass our own and whose generous gifts of vitality and healing enrich our lives and make us whole?

Empowering our patients to adopt a lifestyle that creates a solid foundation for health is an essential beginning. Nutritional habits should include good quality, organic food eaten in a peaceful setting with adequate protein, appropriate fats and carbohydrates, and an abundance of fresh fruits and vegetables. Drinking plenty of fresh clean water, exercising outdoors in the open air and sunshine, getting plenty of restful sleep, and basic hygiene are all essential for health and well-being.

No matter how clean and healthy the house or workplace is kept, the indoor air is always stale compared to the great outdoors. Reclaiming an appreciation for the gifts of each season helps get us outdoors in all seasons, restoring harmony with nature's cycles and in turn, our own natural cycles. What other cure can there be for the current epidemic of "nature deficit disorder" but to step back out into the great outdoors, as often as possible?

Healthy relationships provide an important foundation for healing. Love actually is the greatest power on earth and the lack of it does little to further our well being. Love and appreciation for ourselves are just as vital as being receptive to the love of those around us. Healthy relationships include our connections to our relatives in the natural world where love is ever present, even when human partners, friends, and family are not available.

One of my teachers, Navajo Medicine Woman Annie Kahn, taught us the following affirmation. I often prescribe it for my patients and encourage them to practice it regularly, as if they mean it.

"I am Beautiful!
I am a Child of Mother Earth.
I am a Child of Father Sky.
I am a Child of the Great Spirit.
I am Beautiful!"

Honoring the seasons, the phases of the moon, and the daily rising and setting of the sun with regular ceremony is a very powerful way to reconnect with the natural world. Ceremony and songs create doorways between our human reality and the world of Spirit and Nature. Such practices also have the much needed effect of slowing us down, if only for a moment.

One of the greatest remedies for low grade depression is to welcome the sun each morning, even if our good morning hello must be sent through a cover of clouds or pouring rain. Greetings can range from a simple whispered communication to a song or ceremony. Welcoming and giving thanks for the returning light after each dark night is a wonderful ritual for refueling the subconscious mind and filling the ailing heart with hope and optimism.

Singing and dancing are always welcomed by the nature spirits, and while they certainly do love ancient traditional songs, what is really important is what comes from the heart. Most mornings I sing one of two traditional Native American morning songs, but sometimes another song pops into my heart. The Beatles tune "Here comes the sun…" or "Oh what a beautiful morning!" (Richard Rodgers and Oscar Hammerstein II) are fabulous morning songs to welcome the new day in the absence of more traditional tunes.

Rainy weather is the brunt of so much whining and complaint, but without it we would not last long. Water is essential to life. Singing to the rain, welcoming and giving thanks for the nourishment returned to the Earth from the Sky above lightens our hearts and helps keep us connected and grateful. Arthur Freed had the idea with his timeless song, "Singin' in the Rain."…"What a glorious feeling! I'm happy again!...I'm singin' and dancin' in the rain!"

In modern times, we are assailed by a sea of environmental toxins in amounts unprecedented in human history. Plastics, heavy metals, exhaust fumes, pesticides, chemical fertilizers, medical waste, synthetic colognes, radiation and electro-magnetic fields fill the air we breathe, the food we eat, and the water we drink and bathe in. Identifying the true underlying cause of any individual patient's ill health ultimately means recognizing and addressing our cultural environment and the choices we all make. In the end, we must collectively learn to slow down to a more humane pace of life, and make less toxic choices. We also must reconnect to our roots and rekindle our relationships with the natural world.

Therapeutic Order

"The highest ideal of therapy is to restore health rapidly, gently, permanently; to remove and destroy the whole disease in the shortest, surest, least harmful way, according to clear comprehensive principles."

-Hahnemann, Samuel, "Organon of Medicine,"
Sixth ed., J.P. Tarcher, Inc., 1982; aphorism 2, p. 10

If our ultimate goal is, as Hahnemann says, to bring about the greatest amount of healing in the quickest yet gentlest manner, we need a framework to help guide our treatment choices.

The following pyramid offers one suggestion for prioritizing treatment plans. Each ascending therapeutic intervention rests on the foundation built by those that lie below, so we start at the bottom to create that foundation.

Surgery
Pharmaceuticals
Replacement Therapy
Stimulate the Healing Process
Nourish, Tonify, Support Organs
Establish a Solid Foundation for Health
Identify and Remove Causes of Disease or Obstacles to Cure

We can see from this model that surgery will be most successful and least harmful if the patient has a foundation that allows him to respond optimally. Similarly, the organism will fare better when we use stimulating therapies, such as homeopathy, while simultaneously nourishing and supporting the organs that need to respond once the patient's vitality is mobilized. Ideally we want to employ therapies that offer the least amount of force while providing the greatest amount of healing.

The first two lines form the base of the pyramid and create the foundation for all other therapies. If, for example, the patient with emphysema smokes two packs of cigarettes per day, the cigarettes present an obstacle to cure which must be dealt with at some point for full healing to occur. Likewise, a structural misalignment may need to be corrected before pain and spasm or internal organ dysfunction can be alleviated.

In the second level we see that a solid foundation for achieving and maintaining health is set into place through proper nutrition, exercise, fresh air, sunshine, good relationships, adequate rest, recreation, and purposeful work.

Some patients may not be ready to make the changes this model asks of them and that's OK. Trusting in the healing power of nature includes honoring patient limitations and trusting their processes. Informing patients is vital, but we do them a disservice, and potentially set them up to fail, when we do not acknowledge their limitations and insist they undertake a change they are not yet ready to institute. The most permanent lifestyle changes are usually those that occur slowly over time.

The third line asks us to identify, then nourish and support, affected organ systems. Often simply by nourishing and tonifying specific organs, patients will begin to experience relief. A good example of this is the patient with Hepatitis C. Whatever the symptoms, we know we must choose the appropriate diet, nutrients, herbs and/or glandular therapies that nourish and support both the liver and immune system if we expect our patient to return to optimal health.

The work of the fourth line of the therapeutic pyramid is to stimulate vitality with therapies such as acupuncture, homeopathy, or energy work. The success of these treatments relies upon the foundation of nourishment and support that the underlying levels provide. The model is not linear however, and some patients will not have the energy to change their lifestyles until their vitality is enhanced.

It is not until the fifth line up that we come to replacement therapy. This treatment option comes up most commonly as hormone replacement in menopausal women, hypothyroidism, and the aging male with declining testosterone levels. When a hormone panel from the lab reveals low levels of circulating hormones, the prescribing physician is tempted to write a prescription for hormone replacement. This category sits in the pyramid for good reason, as there certainly are times when replacement therapy is warranted, but not perhaps as often we might suppose.

In menopausal women, restoring optimal function to worn out adrenal glands, tonifying the liver, and in some cases, stimulating vitality, are generally effective in relieving symptoms due to hormone imbalance. The key is to ask ourselves the right questions.

"What is it here that really needs to be healed? Why is the body not able to negotiate its way through what is really a normal life transition? What organs are struggling from toxemia and not able to function adequately and how can I nourish these organs back to optimal function to avoid administering exogenous hormones?"

Low thyroid function responds well to a program that nourishes and restores the gland, but if our patient's hypothyroid condition is due to a significant autoimmune attack on the gland that is initially unresponsive to interventions like discontinuing gluten, it may be necessary to temporarily administer thyroid hormone to the patient until we can realign and heal the underlying immune dysfunction.

Chapter 2

Principles of Homeopathy

"The highest ideal of cure is rapid, gentle, and permanent restoration of health...in the shortest, most reliable, and most harmless way, on easily comprehensible principles."

-Hahnemann, The Organon of Medicine, Sixth ed., Aphorism 2

THESE WORDS WERE WRITTEN in the early 1800's by Dr. Samuel Hahnemann, founder of the system of medicine we now know as homeopathy. Dr. Hahnemann was a physician, chemist, and researcher, who abandoned his highly successful medical practice, because he felt he was doing more harm than good in utilizing the toxic substances and harmful procedures common to the conventional medical practices of his time. Turning to his skills in language, he began translating medical texts and discovered a treatise on the use of Peruvian bark in the treatment of malaria. It was this article that sparked his curiosity, changed his thinking, and eventually led to the development of a whole new system of healing, now known as homeopathy.

MINIMUM DOSE AND THE LAW OF SIMILARS

One of the basic tenets of homeopathic philosophy is the idea that a small dose of a substance will stimulate healing of symptoms that are the same or similar to those caused when a larger dose is taken. The potentially toxic plant, Belladonna, for example, causes a hot flushed face and dilated pupils in overdose. When this same plant is administered in homeopathic dosages, it is highly effective in treating a fever that is accompanied by a hot, flushed face and dilated pupils.

In administering a dilution of a substance that in a material dose causes the very symptoms we desire to cure homeopaths work with the process, acknowledging that the body generates symptoms in an attempt to cure an underlying problem. Minute doses of a well selected remedy enable the body to move through these symptoms. Patient complaints often disappear quickly, not because they have been suppressed, but rather, because the healing process has been supported in such a manner that there is no longer any need for the body to produce symptoms.

The law of similars reminds us of one of the most important tenets of naturopathic medicine, "Vis Medicatrix Naturae", the healing power of nature. Nowhere is the philosophy of honoring and working with the wisdom of the body more present than in the practice of homeopathy.

Potentizing the Homeopathic Remedy

Homeopathic medicines are prepared by a series of dilutions and shaking. The term used in homeopathy to describe the shaking is succussion.

The substance that is to be made into a remedy is first diluted in a concentration of 1:10 or 1:100, and then shaken or succussed vigorously 100 times. One part of this dilution (usually one drop) is then mixed with 9 or 99 parts of water, and again the bottle is succussed vigorously. This process is repeated until the desired potency is achieved.

A medicine that is diluted and succussed at a 1:10 concentration 6 times is a 6X potency. If it is diluted at a 1:100 concentration 30 times, it becomes a 30C potency. The numbers 6 or 30 refer to the number of dilutions and succussions that occur in the process of preparing the medicine. The "X" or "C" that is written after the number indicates the concentration, with "X" being the 1:10, or decimal dilution, and "C" being the 1:100, or centesimal dilution.

The more times that a medicine is diluted and succussed, the stronger it becomes in its ability to affect a healing response in the organism. Although Hahnemann's work preceded the birth of quantum physics by a good century, Einstein's discovery that matter and energy are just two ends of the same continuum helps explain the power of the diluted dose. In the process of potentization, a material substance is taken back to its energetic form, rendering it more energetically potent, despite its increasing lack of physical form.

The substances commonly used to prepare homeopathic remedies originate in nature. Plants, minerals, and animal substances provide the raw material for most of the remedies that are used in everyday practice. Some less common remedies are prepared from diseased tissue. These special remedies are called nosodes.

On an even rarer occasion, a remedy may be made from a pharmaceutical medication. These drug remedies, when prescribed in a low (6, 12 or 30) potency are often very effective at relieving withdrawal symptoms, allowing the patient to discontinue the pharmaceutical drug far more easily.

Withdrawal symptoms are not the same as the symptoms for which the drug was prescribed in the first place. For example, the patient who was prescribed paxil for depression or anxiety who has a return of the same depressive symptoms on stopping the drug is not going through withdrawal. This patient needs to be treated for the original depression and in fact I do not withdraw pharmaceutical medications until I feel assured that the treatment I am using is helping with the original condition.

If, on the other hand, the patient experiences electrical sensations, dizziness, or nausea on withdrawing the drug, then they can be treated with a homeopathic nosode made from the drug. The homeopathic preparation is taken as needed for withdrawal symptoms. This approach has been very effective at helping patients stop medications that might otherwise be very difficult to discontinue.

Remedy Selection

Selection of the homeopathic remedy is very individualized, taking into consideration, not only the diagnosis, but also the individual manifestation of symptoms as they occur in that particular patient. Symptom patterns of the patient are elicited with painstaking detail. Not only does the homeopath want to know that the patient has a cough, but we also need to learn how long the patient has had the cough, if it came on suddenly or gradually, and if there are other symptoms that accompany the cough. What circumstances are likely to alleviate or aggravate the presenting symptom? Is the cough better or worse in certain positions, by changes in weather or at specific times of day? The quality of the symptom is also important. Is the cough harsh, dry and spasmodic, or loose with easy expectoration?

In choosing a homeopathic remedy, we want to know something about the person's emotional state. What is the patient's basic personality? Have there been changes in the patient's emotional responses since becoming ill? What, if any, physical or emotional stresses preceded the onset of symptoms?

Where homeopathic medicines are suggested in this book, the selection of the remedy is generally uncomplicated and fairly straightforward. Many conditions, especially chronic ongoing diseases, require a deep acting "constitutional" remedy which is highly individualized and must be selected by a trained homeopath. Because homeopathy works by stimulating the patient's vitality, it is often highly effective at treating and even healing conditions that are unresponsive to conventional methods.

Repetition of the Dose

Once a patient's vitality is enhanced by administration of a well selected homeopathic remedy, more energy is available to the body for the healing process to take place. It is important to remember however, that it is the patient's own body that does the healing, not the remedy. The homeopathic remedy acts only as a stimulus to mobilize the patient's inherent healing abilities, and because of this, it is usually dosed only as needed. Once a healing reaction has begun, the frequency of repetition is tapered down or discontinued, depending on the degree of response that occurs.

To illustrate this point, let's use the example of riding a horse. When movement is desired, a little leg pressure is applied to urge the horse forward. Once the horse responds, the pressure is released and is not applied again unless the horse threatens to slow down or the rider wants the horse to move faster. Like the pressure of the rider's leg signaling the horse to move forward, a correctly prescribed remedy stimulates the patient's innate healing mechanisms, and just as the horse is the one who does the actual work, it is the patient's own body that does the actual healing. The forward movement may be stimulated by the rider's cue or the homeopathic medicine, but neither of these things do the actual work.

Potency Selection

Homeopathic remedies are commonly available as 6x, 12x, 30x, 6C, 12C, 30C, 200C, 1M, and 10M. The lower numbers are less dilute and not as energetically strong as the higher numbered remedies, which are more dilute and therefore more potent in their ability to stimulate healing. As it is possible to over stimulate the vital force with higher potencies, it is usually recommended that the 6, 12, 30 and 200 potencies be used if you are new to homeopathy.

Generally, for acute conditions a potency of 200C can be dosed every 4 - 8 hours, whereas a 30C may need to be repeated every 2 - 4 hours. While I usually find the 200C potency to be most effective in treating the majority of acute diseases, if a 30C is all that is at hand, it may work just as well.

Potency selection is based on the severity of the condition being treated and the vitality of the patient. The size or age of the patient is really not so much a consideration. A newborn infant or a tiny little kitty may be dosed with a high potency if the illness is very fast paced and intense. A huge full grown elephant with a low grade chronic condition might be treated with a low potency. The same elephant with an acute problem would respond better to the higher potency.

Remedies are most commonly dispensed on sugar pellets of varying sizes. Because the potency has already been determined by the process of dilution and succussion, the exact number of pellets given in any one dose is not critical. Remedies may also be administered in water rather than on pellets.

A good equestrian, in tune with the sensitivity of the horse, will use the least amount of force in cuing the animal. Similarly, the skilled practitioner must assess each patient to determine the least amount of intervention that will bring about the greatest healing in a manner that is gentle, yet rapid and thorough. This concept holds true, not only in selecting the appropriate potency for homeopathic prescribing, but for all our therapies.

In chronic disease, a prescription of a 200C or 1M potency may initially cause an aggravation of symptoms that is usually short lived, lasting perhaps a day or two. Such aggravations are usually mild and and are actually viewed as a positive indication that the correct remedy is working appropriately. This slight increase in symptoms that precedes resolution and healing may be a result of an attempt by the body to rid itself of toxins. Aggravations are rarely seen in acute illness, however, as the body is usually already very actively discharging. In these latter cases, the remedy helps bring resolution of symptoms without aggravation.

LM potencies, utilized by some homeopaths for chronic conditions, are prepared with larger dilutions and less succussion. These potencies are gentle enough to be prescribed for daily use without concern for the possible aggravation of symptoms that may occur when higher potencies are prescribed. The LM potencies are generally my preferred dose for patients struggling with chronic disease.

An exhausted, worn down patient who presents to clinic with a history of multiple losses and grief, poorly controlled diabetes, fatigue, and fullness in the liver may not have as much vitality as a younger, more robust patient who suffers from a chronic sinusitis and occasional insomnia. While the more vital patient with the sinus symptoms may do fine with a 200C or 1M potency, the less vital patient may be better served with a lower potency.

LM potencies may be the perfect place to start with the exhausted diabetic patient struggling with multiple problems, because the LM potency acts as a gentle nudge and will be less likely to over stimulate a patient who is not strong enough to tolerate the possible aggravation that may occur with a higher potency. Unlike higher potencies, which are given only once, the LM doses are usually dispensed in water and repeated once or twice a day for several weeks or months.

In contrast, a younger patient who is strong and active may do fine with a higher potency, such as a 200C or 1M given only once. The potency is selected according to the intensity of the symptoms as well as the sensitivity and vitality of the patient.

Frequency of repetition is dependent partly on the potency that is being used and partly on the severity of the problem. In an acute condition, repetition of a 200C can easily be made every 4 - 8 hours as needed. In a more serious and quickly progressing situation, the remedy is repeated as the symptoms demand, and if the situation is serious enough, it may be necessary to use an even higher potency, like a 10 M, in frequently repeated doses.

Case

A woman comes to the clinic with a bladder infection of recent onset. She describes some burning which is worse after urination, but says her most significant symptom is a sharp cramping pain right after urination. She is given homeopathic Sarsaparilla in a 200C to be repeated every 4 hours for the first 24 hours while she is awake, then every 6 - 8 hours for the second 24 hours, followed by every 6 - 8 hours as needed.

It is essential to impress upon patients the importance of repeating the remedy if symptoms threaten to return, while warning them not to keep repeating the dose endlessly once they are doing better. I have rarely seen a problem with patients taking the correctly prescribed remedy too often when needed in an acute state, but I have certainly witnessed lots of relapses when patients stopped the remedy too soon.

The homeopathic remedy should be discontinued if frequent dosing does not result in significant improvement within the first 24 hours, as this usually implies that the remedy is not the right one for the case. Any worsening of symptoms, should it occur, is usually a sign that the disease is simply progressing. It is rarely a result of remedy repetition, except perhaps in the most sensitive patients.

The administration of herbs with the homeopathic remedy will often serve to initiate healing even when the wrong remedy has been presecribed. While a well selected remedy will usually promote rapid resolution of symptoms in a truly acute condition, the wrong remedy will usually have no effect, wasting valuable healing time if nothing else is offered.

The herbal formula supports the action of the homeopathic remedy by nourishing affected tissues. Fortunately some cases will heal with the herbs alone, although healing is generally more rapid when the correct remedy accompanies herbal prescriptions, and vice versa.

Our patient with the acute bladder infection responded quickly to the homeopathic Sarsaparilla 200C, experiencing significant relief within 15 minutes of taking the first dose. She found she did best if she continued to repeat the remedy every 4 hours for 3 more doses, after which she was able to reduce her repetitions to every 6 - 8 hours. On the third day she took the remedy twice, then once more on the forth day, as just a bit of slight burning suggested her vitality could use another boost.

Despite complete resolution of symptoms, I suggested she continue to take the herbs I had also prescribed, reducing the dose from every 2 - 4 hours to 3 - 4 times per day for 4 -5 more days to provide continued nourishment and support to healing tissues.

The Similimum

Although the practice of homeopathy certainly demands some hard work and study, especially on the part of the beginning practitioner, it does not need to be the overwhelming challenge it is often painted to be by many homeopathic practitioners. The hours of study initially invested in learning homeopathy bring abundant rewards for both practitioner and patient as many "incurable" conditions often respond to the correctly prescribed remedy when all other therapies fail. Yet, sadly too many practitioners, intimidated by perfectionistic insistence on getting the exact "simillimum" or similar remedy, often turn away from relying on homeopathy as a therapeutic modality.

Despite protestations to the contrary by some homeopathic practitioners, many patients respond well to commonly known "polycrests" such as Sepia, Lycopodium, Pulsatilla, Natrum muriaticum, Thuja, Tuberculinum, Medorrhinum, Aurum, and others. Although one could certainly argue that many patients might do better if they received a more specific remedy, as long as the patient's overall health is improving according to the laws of cure - from above down, from within outward, and in reverse order - healing is occurring. Often a polycrest (commonly known remedy) will be close enough to the patient's constitution to provoke a healing reaction.

Nearly all my patients receive constitutional homeopathic medicines, which has appeared to be essential in providing the energetic shift and mobilization of vitality that enables other therapies to work effectively and efficiently.

The following story illustrates a case when the exact remedy made all the difference in a patient who was doing well on a polycrest, but soared when given her simillimum. Had I never found her exact remedy, she would still have been grateful for the enormous amount of healing she received from the polycrest remedy.

Case

Susan, who had been coming to the office for some years, had improved significantly, both emotionally and physically, with periodic prescriptions of homeopathic Sepia. Her irritability, menstrual symptoms, and fatigue were all relieved with the polycrest prescription. Even though the relief was not as long lasting and permanent as I might have liked, the polycrest remedy enabled her to move forward with her life, explore the inner dimensions of her emotional pain, and pursue a career in marketing.

Had Susan not later received the deeper acting remedy, Mandragora, this highly motivated patient would still have continued to progress. Once I learned of Mandragora, however, and prescribed it in a single dose, the results were dramatic and long lasting. This more precise simillimum brought relief to her constant sense of inner torment, and the overriding feeling that her life was cursed, as well as clearing her physical symptoms. The irritability, menstrual complaints, and her general health improved dramatically. Her confidence soared allowing her to move forward in her life in a way that had not been possible before.

Although Sepia was definitely moving her along on the path to health, it was not able to affect her as deeply and quickly as the Mandragora. Life does not always lead us to the one exact remedy that for all we know may not even have been discovered yet. As I often tell my patients, "There is the ideal, and then there is what's real."

All we can do is strive to offer our best effort to each and every patient that seeks our help on their path to wholeness. In the meantime, most patients will benefit more from a well prescribed polycrest than from no remedy at all.

Cell Salts

Cell salts, also known as tissue salts, are low dose homeopathic remedies made from salts of certain minerals that are found in various tissues of the body. These remedies have a particular affinity for healing specific tissues.

There are a total of twelve of these remedies, generally available in health food stores, herb shops, and whole food groceries. They are only dispensed in 6X or 12X potencies, as it is thought that the lower potencies provide an energetic boost to the tissue they nourish. For example, Calc phos (a phosphorus salt of calcium,) might be given for bone healing or as an adjunct in the treatment of osteoporosis, while another cell salt, Kali phos (Kali phosphoricum from potassium phosphate) is specific for the nervous system. Silica may be added in to enhance immune function or bone integrity.

Cell salts can also be used to help aid in absorption and utilization of certain nutrients. Ferrum phos (Ferrum phosphoricum), for example, is often prescribed when iron deficiency is present.

Because these remedies are so low in potency, they may be safely administered over an extended period of time, up to several months if necessary.

Although constitutionally prescribed homeopathic remedies are generally given alone without other homeopathic remedies, cell salts will rarely be a problem if they are added to the patient's protocol when needed. That having been said, the need for a cell salt may be decreased when the correct constitutional remedy is given.

Chapter 3
Herbs That Act as Adrenal Adaptogens

THE WORD ADAPTOGEN, a relatively new term to herbal medicine, was originally coined in 1947 by the Russian scientist N. V. Lazarev. Plants that are classed as adaptogens are generally tonic and restorative to overall health and can usually be taken long term with little to no ill effects. Adaptogenic plants improve our ability to cope with life stressors, physiologically, mentally and emotionally.

This group of herbs works largely by nourishing and normalizing the function of the outer layer of the adrenal glands called the adrenal cortex. The adrenal cortex can become depleted by chronic stress or toxic overload. Unlike the adrenal medulla, which secretes the "fight or flight hormone" adrenaline, the cortex produces hormones that are vital for maintaining electrolyte balance, regulating carbohydrate, protein, and fat metabolism, modulating inflammation, and enhancing our ability to withstand physical and emotional stress. The adrenal cortex also secretes small amounts of reproductive hormones, making it a key player whenever hormonal imbalances are part of the patient picture.

The use of adaptogenic herbs during times of stress results in a decreased incidence of both chronic and acute disease as immune function is optimized and inflammation modulated. Athletic performance and work productivity improve as a result of increased endurance, and improved mental clarity. The quality of sleep is improved and the ability to make decisions and process emotions is also enhanced.

One plant family, Araliaceae, contains several adaptogenic plants, including Siberian Ginseng (Eleutherococcus senticosus), Devil's Club (Oplopanax horridum), Oriental Ginseng (Panax ginseng), American Ginseng (Panax quinquefolius), and Spikenard (Aralia spp.).

Other adaptogenic plants that are not part of the Araliaceae family, include Licorice Root (Glycerrhiza glabra), Cat's Claw (Uncaria tomentosa), Holy Basil (Ocimum sanctum), Gotu Kola (Centella asiatica), Aswaghanda (Withania somnifera), Reishi Mushroom (Ganoderma lucidum), Maca (Lepidium meyenii), and many others.

Because the adrenal cortex plays an important role in modulating inflammation, adaptogenic herbs are often given to patients suffering with chronic inflammation. Arthritis, autoimmune disease, and cardiovascular disease are a few examples of chronic inflammatory conditions that may benefit with the addition of adrenal adaptogens. In addition, adrenal cortical hormones modulate allergic response, suggesting that conditions such as asthma and hay fever should include adaptogens as part of the treatment protocol.

Because the adrenal cortex is responsible for secreting testosterone, estrogen, and progesterone, adaptogens can play a vital role in the treatment of menstrual disorders, menopausal symptoms, libido, and sexual dysfunction. The abnormal hormone panels seen so commonly in clinical practice are often due at least in part to fatigued adrenal glands.

Inclusion of adrenal herbs in the treatment of diabetes or dysglycemia can help normalize blood sugar, as glucose regulating glucocorticoids secreted by the adrenal cortex may not be circulating at optimal levels in the presence of adrenal fatigue.

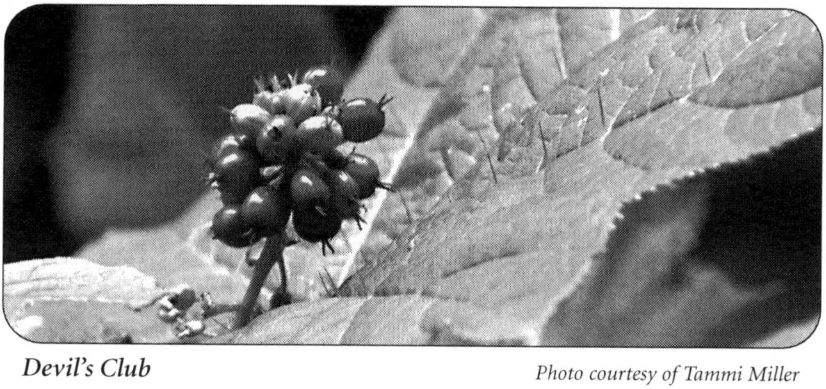

Devil's Club *Photo courtesy of Tammi Miller*

Devil's Club (Oplopanax horridus) Araliaceae

Native to the Pacific Northwest, Oplopanax is most prevalent in moist, shady old growth forests and along stream beds, where it rises to a height of 3 to 10 feet. Its branches reach out in a graceful, majestic fashion with soft leaves that are shaped somewhat like those of a maple tree or thimbleberry bush. In spring, green or whitish flowers can be seen blooming in panicles at the top of each plant, turning to red berries by midsummer. This majestic, no nonsense plant gives the impression of having been here with the dinosaurs. Covered with sharp, spiny, fishhook-like thorns from its base at the earth to the tip of each leaf, this plant has no qualms about protecting itself.

Oplopanax is central to Northwest Native American culture and ceremony where it is viewed as a sacred protective ally as well as a powerful medicine. Historically the plant has been used for arthritis, rheumatism, and respiratory conditions and in large doses as a cleansing purgative and emetic.

In lingering respiratory conditions, Oplopanax is particularly useful for those dry, nonproductive, hacking coughs that seem to nag at the patient long after symptoms should have resolved. In these cases, Oplopanax acts as an expectorant, empowering the cough to fruitfulness and bringing final resolution to the problem.

Traditionally, a poultice has been used topically for various skin conditions and for the treatment of infected wounds and snakebite. The root bark is used in medicine and doses of 60 drops three times per day have been used for the treatment of mild to moderate non-insulin dependent diabetes.

As a protective warrior herb, Oplopanax is well indicated for those meek overly nice souls who are easily overpowered in the face of adversity or for those folks who express a desire to reclaim their power but cannot seem to do so, either from fear, or the toxic overlay of family or cultural taboo.

In cases of acute anxiety, a few drops of Oplopanax tincture can be added to a bottle of the traditional Bach flower essence formula, Rescue Remedy, where it invariably serves to potentize the formula. Rescue Remedy is specifically indicated for panic, shock, and acute anxiety. The addition of Oplopanax compliments the calming and grounding qualities of the flower essence by empowering the patient to stand strong in the face of adversity. Patients report needing less frequent dosing of the Rescue Remedy when Oplopanax is added. One woman described the empowering qualities of the herb perfectly when she shared her experience.

"You know the straight Rescue Remedy does calm me and take away the feeling of panic, but with the addition of that herb

(Oplopanax), I find myself saying, 'What's wrong with me?! I have the power to deal with this!'"

Positive integration of the warrior archetype enables us to stand up for ourselves and set boundaries, effectively, appropriately, and even fiercely when circumstances demand. Whether the demons we must face come from within or without, Oplopanax can be an invaluable ally in the process of integrating personal power.

Although Oplopanax can be found from the Northwestern United States, up into British Columbia and Alaska, its habitat of wetlands and old growth forests is endangered. For this reason, it may be best to use this plant for specific indications only and then only in drop doses to synergize a formula and empower the patient's journey to health and wholeness.

Spikenard (Aralia spp.) Araliaceae

As we move south from the Northwest into Southern Oregon and Northern California, Oplopanax begins to thin out and disappear as another adaptogen, more suited to the drier landscape, emerges to take its place.

Aralia californica is soft and friendly in appearance, lacking the multitude of spines that cause one to stand back from Oplopanax. In fact the inviting beauty of Aralia seems to welcome us closer, as if her inner strength is sufficient to handle whatever comes her way. This gentle grandmother enables us to trust our boundaries and inner resources enough to open up and be receptive to life and the relationships it offers, with all their ups and downs. Delight is the word that comes to mind whenever I encounter Aralia in the wild or as a medicine. Many experience her energy as uplifting and even a bit playful, especially in comparison to the more serious grandfatherly Oplopanax.

In addition to its use as an adaptogen, Aralia may be used for dry or moist coughs, where it acts to soothe inflamed mucous membranes, enhance expectoration and lend anti-microbial properties. It is well indicated for allergic and asthmatic coughs, repeating the theme of relaxing and allowing things in, instead of reacting and closing down. Another herbalist recently shared that she finds Aralia berries helpful in alleviating depression.

Other species include Aralia nudicalis and the more commonly known Aralia racemosa.

The roots are generally harvested for medicine, although berries and leaves have also been used.

Oriental Ginseng (Panax ginseng) and American Ginseng (Panax quinquefolius) Araliaceae

Like other adaptogens, the root of Panax spp. increases stamina, decreases inflammation and tendency to infection, and enables us to handle stressors more effectively. This plant is hepato-protective, antiviral, and may increase levels of interferon. Panax has been used in the treatment of cancer, where it appears to act both as an anti-tumor agent as well as aiding to mitigate side effects from treatment with radiation.

In Asia, Ginseng is considered specific for elders. Recent research indicating usefulness in treating memory loss, decreasing cognitive function, and cerebral ischemia validate this traditional use[1]. Like many other adaptogens it has also been found useful for the treatment of erectile dysfunction, another symptom associated with aging. In addition, optimization of cholesterol levels may be seen[2].

In diabetes, ginseng aids in reducing blood sugar levels by stimulating increased secretion of insulin from the pancreas and enhancing cell uptake of insulin[3].

The Panax ginsengs can be overstimulating and should be avoided in patients who are feeling high strung, restless, and nervous, often referred to as "wired tired." Instead, this adaptogen may find better use for patients who are struggling with lethargy, fatigue, and weakness.

Ginseng appears to act as a tonic to the adrenal cortex, where it has been shown to normalize cortisol levels. While other adaptogens may work just as well, Panax is one of the few adaptogens where research has shown safety and efficacy in the treatment of Cushing's Syndrome, a condition where abnormally increased adreno-cortical function results in chronically elevated levels of cortisol. Many animals, especially horses, but also some dogs, suffer from Cushing's Syndrome. The adaptogenic Chinese herb Gynostemma pentaphylum may also be considered for these cases. Licorice is contraindicated in these cases.

Panax is treasured both here in the United States and in Asia. However the plant has been over harvested on both continents so use of another adaptogen may be best unless this one seems very specifically indicated. Dosage of a 1:1 fresh or 1:4 dry root (Tilgner) tincture is 30 - 60 drops 3 - 4 times daily. Tea may be prepared by decocting 1 teaspoon per cup of water with only the slightest simmer. Alternatively, the root may be infused for 20 - 30 minutes.

The American ginseng is less warming than its Asian cousin.

Siberian Ginseng (Eleutherococcus senticosus) Araliaceae

Eleutherococcus is an invaluable ally in enhancing physiological responses to stress. Repeated studies show that the quality and quantity of work performance is enhanced when Eleutherococcus is taken on a regular basis for a period of time. General resistance to disease is improved with fewer incidences of influenza and other illnesses. Patients exhibiting symptoms of irritability, anxiety, insomnia, or general exhaustion experience an increased sense of well-being, feel less fatigued and are more able to relax. Other studies reveal enhanced physical endurance in athletes, including horses, with an increased ability to handle cold weather. Eleutherococcus can also be of assistance in normalization of blood sugar.

Unlike its relatives in the Panax genus, (Oriental and American ginsengs) Eleutherococcus does not over stimulate. There is some reference to the plant being contraindicated in hypertension[4], however I have used it unwittingly for years in hypertensive patients without ill effects. Another study published in 2004[5] showed positive results in mental and social functioning in twenty hypertensive patients over the age of 65 who were also receiving digitalis, a heart medication whose toxicity is easily potentiated by a multitude of substances. The use of Eleutherococcus, did not demonstrate any deleterious change in blood pressure control and no digitalis toxicity occurred over the period of eight weeks that the study was done.

Ashwaghanda (Withania somnifera) Solanaceae

Leaving the Araliaceae family, we move to Withania, an ayurvedic herb from India. Like the adaptogens generally, it is well indicated in cases of nervous exhaustion, where stress and strain have wrecked havoc on overwrought nerves, further exacerbating the problem by leaving the patient in a sleepless state of nervous unrest.

Dr. Vasant Ladd ("The Yoga of Herbs,") tells us that Ashwaghanda "has the smell of a horse, (and) gives the vitality and sexual energy of a horse."

One can only presume that Dr. Ladd is referring to a stallion. Although probably most any adaptogen, with the exception of Glycerrhiza, can be used effectively for treating low libido and waning erectile function, some herbs such as Maca and Ashwaghanda have more reputation for helping with these conditions.

Aswaghanda has been shown to enhance thyroid function resulting in increased levels of thyroid hormones T4 and possibly T3 although other studies do not corroborate the increase in T3[6].

Like most adaptogens, ashwaghanda is anti-inflammatory and supportive to immune function. It has nutritive and anti-oxidant activity and has been shown to reduce lipid peroxidation in the liver while increasing the activity of anti-oxidant enzymes, superoxide dismutase and catalase[7].

Ashwaghanda been used as an adjunct in the treatment of cancer and cachexia. It is calming to the central nervous system as well as restorative to adreno-cortical function.

The root is used in medicine.

A group of us sat with ashwaghanda for a while one evening then shared our experiences. One of the herbalists reported feeling a joyous desire to dance and break free from the bondage of the many rules, cultural morays, taboos, and dogmas that threaten to suppress our vitality and zest for life into a drab existence of meaningless servitude. Another group member said she felt as if the herb could clear a tendency to tear ourselves apart with self criticism and condemnation, while yet another said it opened his crown chakra, conveying a feeling of expansion combined with a deep sense of comfort in the face of the vastness of the universe. The last herbalist shared that the plant "played hide and seek" with him in a playful, lighthearted way causing him to feel giddy with joy. The plant is well indicated for patients who feel trapped.

Powdered herb can be dosed at 10 grams per day taken in divided doses. A reasonable dose of 1:1 fresh plant tincture runs from 30 - 60 drops 3 - 4 times daily.

Cat's Claw (Uncaria tomentosa) Rubiaceae

Cat's claw, native to Peru, is rich in a multitude of bioactive constituents, including a variety of flavonoids, glycosides, and alkaloids, giving the plant significant health benefits that serve to enhance its adaptogenic activities. Flavonoids such as quercitin lend additional anti-allergic activity, while other flavonoids increase anti-inflammatory and anti-oxidant activities of the plant. Catechin, a specific type of flavonoid found in cat's claw, is a constituent that is generally thought to lend hepato-protective as well as anti-oxidant activity[8,9].

Some of the alkaloids present in cat's claw are thought to be responsible for immune enhancing, anti-microbial, anti-viral, and anti-cancer activity. The herb has also been shown to be somewhat anti-hypertensive, and anti-arthritic. It is reputed to be particularly useful for correcting menstrual and hormonal irregularities in women as well as increasing waning libido. Other constituents that may be of interest include beta sitosterol and campesterol, two plant sterols that may be of use in reducing elevated cholesterol.

Cat's claw has astringent qualities, which can help tighten up boggy mucous membranes, including those of the gastro-intestinal tract. Chronic or acute diarrhea, for example, may be helped by the addition of astringent herbs. Because astringent herbs help reduce bleeding, they can be of use in conditions such as ulcerative colitis, especially when the patient has a tendency to blood in the stool.

Astringency also helps tighten leaky mucous membranes of the respiratory and genito-urinary tracts, where it may prove useful for sinus infections, loose coughs with an oversecretion of mucous (most coughs are too dry), menorrhagia (hemorrhagic menses), and vaginal or urethral catarrh.

Many practitioners report good results using cat's claw for the treatment of autoimmune conditions, favoring it over other adaptogenic herbs in these cases. It seems to be a particularly helpful adaptogen for the treatment of Lyme disease. One herbalist prescribed a high dose of 5000 milligrams twice daily for a patient with significant neurological symptoms associated with Lyme disease. The patient experienced significant relief with each dose but reported that the positive effects wore off after 6 hours. She found more consistent relief when the dose was altered to 2500 mg. every 6 hours.

Cat's claw is named for the thorns that extrude from the vine and resemble the claws of a cat. Bark, roots, and leaves are all utilized for medicine. The herb is safe to prescribe in high doses.

Dried powdered herb may be given as high as 10 grams per day, as was done with the Lyme's patient mentioned above. While this higher dosing will be more efficacious in severe Lyme disease, 1 to 4 grams per day, given in divided doses will usually be sufficient for most folks.

Please understand that Lyme disease doesn't easily respond to any one herb and often requires frequent rotation of herbal prescriptions.

Gotu Kola (Centella asiatica) Umbelliferae

Gotu kola, another adaptogen from India, has a special affinity for regenerating the brain and central nervous system, as well as modulating adrenal cortical function, making it more specific for patients with mental fogginess, decreased mental clarity, and difficulty in concentrating. It is one of the primary herbs to consider for cognitive difficulties at any age.

Scientific research suggests that gotu kola may be effective in enhancing healthy connective tissue growth and regeneration in the body, thus preventing the formation of excessive or abnormal scar tissue, and possibly preventing fibrosis[10]. Regular use of gotu kola in inflammatory liver disease, for example, may delay or prevent the development of cirrhosis.[11]

Gotu kola is traditionally classed as a blood cleanser, suggesting that it may be a helpful adjunct in alleviating the stress of toxemia. Because this plant is rich in minerals, I prefer to dose it as a powder or in capsules with 250 - 500 milligrams per day being an average dose. Minerals will also extract in a vinegar extract or to a lesser extent in tea. Although the tincture is quite efficacious for many of the herb's medicinal qualities, the minerals will not be extracted into an alcoholic preparation. The tea is delicious and can be prepared by infusing 1 tablespoonful of herb into each cup of water. When tincture is used a 1:1 preparation made from fresh leaves can be dosed at 60 drops 4 times per day.

Holy Basil, Tulsi
(Ocimum sanctum) Lamiaceae

Holy basil is closely related to the more commonly known sweet basil (Ocimum basilicum). Both plants originally hail from India and both are used as culinary herbs, but holy basil adds a hot peppery spiciness to its aromatics that sweet basil lacks.

In addition to being an excellent adaptogen, holy basil has been shown to be anti-inflammatory, modulating prostaglandin, leukotriene and arachadonic acid metabolism as well as inhibiting COX 2 enzyme systems.[12] Several studies suggest that holy basil may be helpful in the treatment of cancer and in protecting from the oxidative effects of radiation.[13]

Holy Basil's anti-allergic and anti-histamine properties combine well with its anti-microbial and immune enhancing activities in the treatment of asthma.

Holy basil is both hepato-protective and anti-viral, making it an exceptional choice for the treatment of viral hepatitis.[14] Glycerrhiza, Schisandra, Centella, and Uncaria are other adaptogenic herbs that should be considered for viral hepatitis.

Several studies confirm that the plant has the ability to aid in normalizing blood sugar in mild to moderate NIDDM (non-insulin dependent diabetes mellitus).[15]

Holy basil has been shown to be of service in the treatment of gastric ulcer.[16] Topical applications have been used to treat ringworm, illustrating its value as an anti-fungal agent.

As an adaptogen, holy basil helps normalize cortisol levels and decrease adrenal hypertrophy.[17] Although the leaves are most commonly employed for medicine, seeds and stem have also been used.

Traditional use in India includes the treatment of bites from poisonous snakes and scorpions. Here it will combine well it with Echinacea, a Native American plant with similar traditional application. The herb should be applied topically as well as taken internally. It goes without saying that some venomous bites are worse than others and professional medical attention should not be neglected in these cases.

Holy basil imparts a sweet, uplifting sensation that makes it a favorite among those who have dabbled with it as a simple. Sacred to Hindu tradition, it is often found planted around sacred shrines. Woody stems may be fashioned into beads to be worn for spiritual protection or for use in prayer and meditation. The common name Tulsi translates to mean "the incomparable one."

Licorice Root (Glycerrhiza glabra) Fabaceae

Licorice root has been shown to prolong the half life of the adrenal stress hormone, cortisol, making it invaluable in treating chronic stress, chronic inflammation, or in helping reduce or discontinue pharmaceutical steroid medications.

As a moisturizing, mucilaginous, demulcent, licorice is indicated whenever mucous membrane inflammation and irritation are present.

Gastro-esophageal reflux, gastritis, inflammatory bowel disease, or ulceration of the gastro-intestinal tract may all be aided by the addition of Glycerrhiza.

Respiratory complaints also respond well to the mucilaginous qualities of licorice. The plant's anti-viral, anti-bacterial, and expectorant properties are also of use in respiratory conditions.

Glycerrhiza contains flavonoids, isoflavones, and phenolic compounds which contribute to its impressive list of medicinal properties. The herb is anti-oxidant, hepato-protective, hormone modulating, estrogenic, anti-mutagenic, anti-allergic, anti-bacterial, and antiviral.

As a yin tonic, licorice has been shown to decrease testosterone levels over the long term, making it a consideration for treating women with hirsutism (abnormal hair growth) and polycystic ovarian syndrome, where testosterone levels are often seen to be elevated.[18] The herb's tendency to lower testosterone makes it an inappropriate choice for the treatment of erectile dysfunction however.

It is also contraindicated in patients with a tendency to fluid retention, hypertension, or in Cushing's syndrome, where elevated cortisol levels are present as a result of an overactive adrenal cortex. While this latter condition is not as common among humans, it is a frequent finding in animals, including horses and to a lesser extent dogs.

Licorice should not be used for patients who are taking cardiac glycosides as its tendency to deplete potassium over the long term may precipitate toxicity reactions from cardio-active glycosides, such as those present in digitalis and its synthetic derivatives.

Like other adaptogenic herbs, licorice increases endurance, stamina and overall well being during times of stress. It is frequently used for the treatment of chronic and acute viral diseases where its actions as an anti-viral, adrenal adaptogen and hepato-protective agent often prove invaluable. For herpes outbreaks, licorice may be used topically as well as internally.

A tincture of 1:3 dried root may be dosed 30 - 60 drops 3 - 4 times per day. Although the root is ideally decocted at 1 teaspoon per cup of water for optimal extraction of medicinal constituents, it is often simply infused and used as a beverage.

Licorice combines well with equal parts of chamomile, fennel seed, and peppermint for use as a tea to alleviate inflammation, gas, and spasm in the intestinal tract.

Maca (Lepidium meyenii) Brassicaceae

Maca hails from the Andes mountains of Peru where it manages to thrive despite severe winters, intense sunlight, and violent winds. A member of the cabbage family, which contains a number of common vegetables, including broccoli, cauliflower, and cabbage, maca is high in nutritious proteins, fats, sugars, starches and minerals, including iodine, calcium, and iron. Due to its rich nutritional content, maca has long been used as a food by the mountain people of Peru.

Maca is rich in sterols, and contains tannins, alkaloids, and saponins. The sterols and saponins combine to give the plant its significant ability to modulate hormones. Recent studies have demonstrated improved sperm quality[19] and quantity when the root was added to cattle feed.

Traditional people did not need modern science to illustrate these properties, however, and so it is that maca has been especially prized over the centuries for its ability to enhance fertility, and improve libido and erectile function. Maca has also been used for menstrual and hormonal irregularities and imbalances, and will aid in improving mental clarity, concentration, physical stamina, and general resistance to disease.

The roots of maca, which are used in both food and medicine, have a delicious malty taste that is guaranteed to enhance any chocolate treat.

Although raw Maca is used in medicine, roasted maca is available as a tasty coffee substitute. Roasting increases stimulating properties of the herb, but is said not to cause the let down and withdrawal symptoms that are associated with coffee.

Due to generally increasing popularity and the harsh climate of its natural habitat, wild crafted maca should not be used. Utilization of farmed maca supports Peruvian farmers and prevents over harvesting and possible extinction of this valuable and delicious plant.

Reishi Mushroom (Ganoderma lucidum) Ganodermataceae

Constituents of this adaptogenic mushroom include polysaccharides, beta-d-glucans, alkaloids, lactones, amino acids, triterpenes, hormonally active sterols, and beta-sitosterol.[20]

As an immune modulator, reishi mushroom is valuable for a wide spectrum of problems ranging from inflammation and allergy to cancer and infectious disease. It is anti-viral, anti-bacterial, anti-histamine, and may help in mitigation of hypersensitivity reactions.[21] Modulation of IgG, IgE, IgA and IgM antibodies suggest the plant may be useful in food sensitivities. Reishi can be utilized for treating duodenal and gastric ulcer inflammation as well as in mitigating food sensitivity reactions due to intestinal permeability syndrome.

Anti-microbial and anti-inflammatory actions extend their usefulness to the respiratory tract, where reishi demonstrates additional activity as an expectorant. Asthmatic patients may find relief due to anti-allergic properties of the plant.

As an anti-oxidant and hepatoprotective herb, reishi can be helpful in enhancing and protecting liver function. The plant has found use in nephritis as well as hepatitis, and like many adaptogens, reishi can be useful in normalizing blood sugar dysregulation.

Reishi may also act as a cardio-vascular tonic. Here it may be useful in formulas to address palpitations, dyspnea, angina, and the edema associated with congestive heart failure. Elevated LDL, triglycerides, and total cholesterol may be corrected through the use of reishi, while beneficial HDL levels have been shown to increase.[22] Cholesterol lowering appears to happen by a decreased synthesis of cholesterol in the liver, another indication of reishi's tonifying effects on that organ. The plant also aids in decreasing elevated blood pressure and normalizing platelet aggregation.[23]

Folks traveling to high mountain elevations may find that the use of Ganoderma, started 10 -14 days before embarking on the journey, will prevent altitude sickness by oxygenating the blood. Ginkgo biloba may be combined with reishi to further potentiate positive effects.

Immune modulating, anti-oxidant, and enhanced liver detoxification actions of this plant contribute to its anti-tumor activity.[24,25] Ganoderma may also be of benefit in enhancing anti-cancer effects of radiation therapy while offering protection from the negative effects.[26,27] Not coincidentally, reishi has been used topically as a sun screen. It may also aid in regenerating bone marrow and spleen.

The Latin species name "lucidum" describes the shiny fruiting body of the mushroom. Traditional Chinese names translate to mean "plant of immortality" and "herb of spiritual potency." It has been used in Asia to ward off evil influences.

Reishi is most commonly found growing on the sides of trees, preferably oaks, and can be found in the United States on the east coast and in the southwest along the gulf coast. It also grows in Europe and South America as well as Asia. It has a tendency to destroy the wood of the tree it feeds on. Cultivated species are preferred as reishi is not common in the wild.

Rhodiola (Rhodiola rosea) Crassulaceae

Rhodiola is another highly effective adaptogen from Russia. Constituents from roots and rhizomes include flavonoids, proanthocyanadins, monoterpene alcohols and their glycosides, cyanogenic glycosides and other glycosides. The presence of flavonoids lends antioxidant properties and combines with adaptogenic actions to enhance anti-inflammatory activity.

Like any adaptogen, Rhodiola helps to reduce fatigue and increase stamina and resistance to disease. It has been shown to alleviate mild to moderate depression, reduce anxiety, and improve concentration and cognitive function.[28] The plant is neuroprotective and cardioprotective, and is reputed to increase life span. There are a number of interesting studies suggesting it to be a helpful adjunct in the treatment of cancer. Another species (R. algida) has been shown to reduce side effects of chemotherapy induced oral mucositis in patients being treated for breast cancer.[29]

I have always felt Rhodiola to be a soothing and strengthening herb for the heart, both emotionally and physically. Although I never had more to go on than a bit of intuition, I often included it in formulas for patients struggling with heartache, sadness, or grief.

I was delighted when Dr. Michael Knapp N.D., shared an abstract from a Russian journal showing that Rhodiola appears to be both cardioprotective and antiarrthymic.[30]

During a myocardial infarction (heart attack), one of the coronary arteries which supply blood to the heart is occluded for a long enough period of time that the portion of the myocardium (heart muscle) that relies on that source of blood dies. The tissue surrounding the point of infarct (tissue death) becomes electrically hypersensitive and begins firing impulses which then cause arrhythmias. Depending on how often and in what patterns they occur, some of these arrhythmias can be deadly in the first days of recovery from a myocardial infarction. Much of what happens in a coronary care unit post infarct is aimed towards preventing these aberrant contractions. According to this study, Rhodiola was seen to "abolish" this electrical instability in the affected areas. It also appears to minimize the amount of tissue death expected to occur as a result of decreased coronary perfusion. Although treatment with Rhodiola can certainly be instituted immediately after an infarct, full effects were not seen for 5 to 8 days in the study, suggesting it may do its best work in the patient who has been on it for at least a week prior to infarct.[31]

The study also suggested that stress induced arrhythmias may also be reduced with the use of Rhodiola.

Although this study was done on rats, and needs to be corroborated in human studies, the benefit of herbal medicine is that we will not do any harm by including Rhodiola in formulas for patients who are at risk for a coronary event.

Suma or Brazilian Ginseng (Pfaffia paniculata) Amaranthaceae

Indigenous to the tropics of South America and the Amazon River Basin, this sizable, sprawling vine is commonly known in Portugese as "para toda" which translates to mean "for all things." Like most adaptogens, it does indeed improve overall health, energy, stamina, and immune function. In South America it is considered a general tonic for many organ systems. It acts on the central nervous system to help soothe and calm overwrought nerves. As a cardiovascular tonic, it aids to regulate blood pressure and reduce atherosclerosis. High levels of germanium in the roots lend an ability to improve oxygenation of the blood.

As with most adaptogens, reproductive tract function is enhanced by the use of Pfaffia. Symptoms of hormonal imbalances such as PMS, menopausal symptoms, low libido, infertility, and erectile dysfunction may all be aided by the addition of Pfaffia.

Pfaffia is regulatory to blood sugar, tonic to digestive functioning, anti-inflammatory in arthritis and rheumatism, and has been used in the treatment of bronchitis. It is also another adaptogen to consider in the treatment of cancer patients.[32,33]

In addition to a large number of saponins, Pffafia contains sitosterol and stigmasterol, which are two constituents thought to be responsible for modulation of reproductive hormones, including estrogen progesterone, and testosterone.[34,35] Nortriterpenes and glycosides are also present.

The plant is highly nutritious consisting of several amino acids, vitamins, electrolytes, and trace minerals, including vitamins B1, B2 and B5, E and K, iron, zinc, magnesium and silica. The presence of iron makes it a good adaptogen to consider for iron deficiency anemia, and may be an herb to consider in the treatment of menorrhagia.

Dosing Adaptogenic Herbs

Adaptogens do well when dispensed in powder for those patients who are willing to take them in that form. Gotu kola is high in minerals which are not well extracted into alcohol, making powdered herb a better choice when minerals are desired. The same goes for Maca, which is quite tasty as well as rich in nutrients.

I usually start patients out on one teaspoon of powdered herb three times per day. For the occasional patient who needs higher dosing, two to four herbs may be mixed together in the powder to be dispensed at double the dose.

Teas of gotu kola, holy basil, and licorice are readily available on the market and may used as a beverage to augment tincture or powder.

Licorice is the one adaptogen that does not do well as a powder as the taste is so strong it tends to overwhelm the palate. Powdered herbs will retain their potency for up to six months after which they should be discarded. Since adaptogens are so frequently needed in a busy practice, powdered herbs will usually be off the shelf in plenty of time.

Tinctures should be dosed at 30 to 60 drops three times daily. Most patients will need at least 60 drops three times per day, although some more seriously depleted folks may need up to 4 teaspoons per day. One can easily see how these patients are underserved when we add one or two adaptogens to a formula and dispense a total of 30 - 60 drops of the entire formula 3 - 4 times daily. Again in higher dosing, it may be wisest to combine 3 - 4 herbs so no single herb is overdosed, although most of these herbs are fine dosed at 60 drops 3 - 4 times daily.

Practitioners often try to dose adaptogens early in the day with the aim of following the body's natural cortisol rhythms. Some patients who do well on adaptogens during the day do notice difficulty in falling asleep if the herbs are taken near bedtime, suggesting that earlier dosing may be preferable. When prescribing in this manner, the adaptogenic herbs may be given in two doses, the first in the morning and the second at noon, although many patients will do fine if the last dose is taken by 3 - 5 PM. For those patients who need additional support for sleep issues a formula of sedative, nervine herbs can be given at bedtime.

Teas of gotu kola, holy basil, and licorice are readily available on the market and may used as a beverage to augment tincture or powder.

Chapter 4

Herbs that Act as Nervines

WHILE ADAPTOGENS CALM by nourishing and restoring the adrenal cortex, nervines soothe by feeding and rebuilding the nervous system. Because these plants work by healing and nourishing overwrought nerves, they are best given regularly whenever symptoms of anxiety, tension, or insomnia are present. Ongoing use of nervines help to nourish and rebuild a strained nervous system, thereby reducing and preventing anxiety, improving sleep, and relieving overall feelings of tension. Many of these herbs also act to alleviate musculo-skeletal spasm. While extra doses may be added as needed for moments when anxiety threatens to erupt, or in anticipation of potentially stressful events, regular dosing is essential to address underlying nervous system dysfunction.

An ideal method for dosing nervines is to take small quantities throughout the day. This can easily be done by making one quart of a strong infusion of loose, dried herbs or by adding 2 or more teaspoons of tincture to a quart of boiling water, allowing it to cool, then sipping it throughout the day.

Nervines combine well with adaptogens, synergistically enhancing the overall effects of each class of herbs.

California Poppy (Eschscholzia californica) Papaveraceae

This beautiful plant, indigenous to western North America, is a member of the poppy family. Although used as a mild analgesic, and musculoskeletal and visceral anti-spasmodic, California poppy lacks the intense opiate alkaloids of its relative, the Opium poppy. Once in bloom, the whole plant is harvested for use as medicine. It is highly effective as a nervine, yet mild enough to use for children or sensitive patients. It can be helpful for intestinal colic or uterine cramps associated with menses, or in a formula for musculoskeletal spasm.

The standard adult dose of a 1:1 fresh plant tincture ranges from 20 to 60 drops up to 4 times per day.

Alkaloids contained in the plant have been shown to have some degree of antifungal activity.[36]

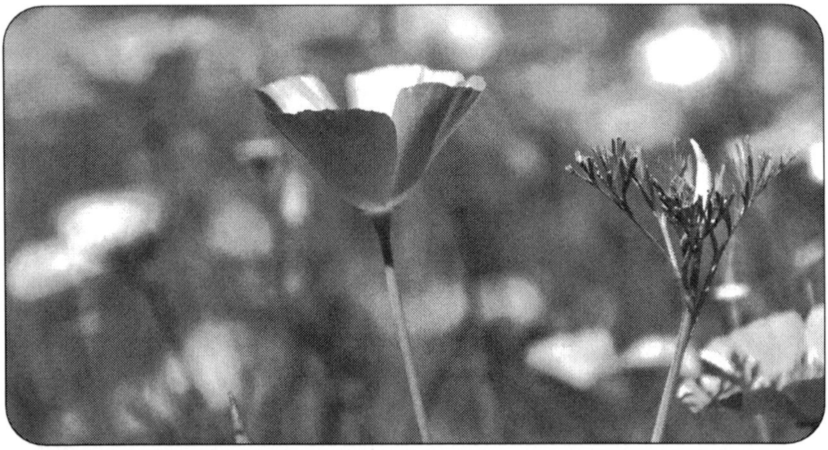

California Poppy *Photo courtesy of Tammi Miller*

Although I have found no references to support the use of California poppy in the treatment of mild to moderate depression, I have personally found it to be uplifting when taken internally. The mere sight of the beautiful, brightly colored orange and yellow flowers is enough to lighten the heavy heart.

Catnip (Nepeta cataria) Laminaceae

Like most members of the mint family, catnip is a carminative, an herb that reduces intestinal colic and gas by enhancing digestion. Essential oils, abundant in the mint family, are often the constituents that provide carminative actions. With catnip, intestinal antispasmodic activity adds to its carminative properties to further reduce pain and discomfort associated with colic. A mild but effective nervine, catnip is safe for babies and children, to soothe ruffled nerves, upset bellies, or both.

Catnip also has emmenogogue activity and may be considered as part of a formula for amenorrhea. Although I would not expect it to work alone in complicated cases, it may bring on menses that are delayed due to stress or digestive upset.

The plant may be administered liberally with the average adult dose being up to 60 drops four times daily of a 1:1 fresh and dry tincture. A tea may be made using 1-2 teaspoons of herb per cup of water then drinking 2 - 4 cups per day.

Chamomile (Matricaria recutita) Asteraceae

The simple chamomile, familiar to most folks, is specifically indicated when nervous tension manifests with restlessness, irritability and oversensitivity to pain. Children who need chamomile will be argumentative and difficult to please, demanding whatever they feel they need in the moment, then unhappily and often quite irritably rejecting it when it is given to them. Their nervous, oversensitive condition causes them to be fidgety and more likely to throw tantrums and scream in displeasure. For these folks, adult or pediatric, chamomile is the nervine of choice, especially when digestive complaints accompany the picture.

Homeopathic preparations of Chamomile are commonly used for the treatment of acute otitis media (middle ear infection) when the same symptoms of oversensitivity and irritable restlessness are present.

Pulsatilla and Belladonna are also common remedies for otitis media unless the child's constitutional remedy is indicated instead. The little one who needs homeopathic Pulsatilla will be only mildly irritable, weepy, whiny and clingy, and less prone to tantrums. Belladonna is more indicated when ear pain comes on suddenly and is accompanied by fever and hot dry skin.

As an herbal tea or tincture, chamomile is anti-inflammatory, anti-spasmodic, and carminative, helping to release and prevent the formation of gas in the digestive tract. It may also be used as part of a protocol to alleviate inflammation in ulcerative colitis, gastritis, or gastric ulcer. Antispasmodic activities bring relief to symptoms of cramping in the bowel, and may again be useful for ulcerative colitis, irritable bowel syndrome, or a simple episode of intestinal gas and spasm. It is helpful for the occasional dyspepsia or nervous stomach, where it works to soothe nerves and digestion both.

The constituent alpha bisabolol makes up a good 50% of the essential oil of the plant and has been credited with much of the anti-inflammatory and anti-spasmodic action of the herb, while chamazulene, a constituent also present in yarrow, adds more anti-inflammatory properties, working at least in part, through inhibition of leuko-triene synthesis.[37] Chamazulene also acts as an anti-oxidant.

Chamomile has anti-allergic, anti-fungal, anti-bacterial, and anti-pyretic activities as well. It can be used topically as an antiseptic and soothing anti-inflammatory agent.

The herb may be dosed liberally and is often preferred as a tea. Infusions can be prepared using from 1 teaspoon to 1 tablespoon of dried herb per cup of water and then drinking as desired. Tincture of a 1:1.5 combination of fresh and dried herb can be taken at 75 drops up to four times daily.

Hops (Humulus lupulus) Cannabaceae

Hops are prized for making beer. The herb grows as a large climbing dioecious vine with male and female reproductive flowers occurring on different plants.

Rich in bitters, hops stimulates digestive juices, while its volatile oils add a carminative action that aids to reduce spasmodic colic in the intestines. Xanthohumoral, a chalcone constituent found in hops, has been shown to be anti-inflammatory and protective to the liver, helping to prevent fibrosis in chronic hepatitis.[38] (Silybum marianum and Centella asiatica should also be considered for the prevention of fibrosis in inflammatory liver disease.)

Xanthohumol contained in hops has also been shown to be anti-cancer,[39] a property further enhanced by the presence of proantho-cyanadins and other flavonoids.

In the reproductive sphere, constituents present in the plant promote healthy estrogen metabolism affecting to a lesser extent progesterone.[40] Hops may be a plant to consider for women going through menopause who are experiencing liver congestion, digestive symptoms, anxiety and insomnia.

Phytoestrogenic compounds in hops and many other plants require healthy intestinal flora to convert plant constituents to biochemically active compounds in the human body. For this reason, probiotics should be considered if digestive symptoms are present or there is any recent history of anti-biotic use or prolonged stress.

Antispasmodic properties of hops are active in the uterus as well as the intestinal tract, making the plant potentially useful for the treatment of dysmenorrhea (menstrual cramps). In these cases hops does its best work if taken early at the first sign of painful spasm.

Traditional folklore suggests that hops may act as an anaphrodisiac in men, decreasing libido and sexual activity. This action has been confirmed by modern science in animal studies.[41]

Although not usually thought of as an immune modulator hops does have some anti-microbial and anti-bacterial activity.

For insomnia hops can be very effective for some folks when used as a dream pillow. Volatile oils inhaled through the nose stimulate the olfactory nerve, which in turn activates the limbic system, a deep, emotional part of the old brain. Hops' soothing volatile oils have a sedative effect on an overstimulated limbic system, allowing sleep.

As a nervine, hops are most specific for the overly intellectualized patient with cerebral congestion preventing sleep. These patients will take their troubles into their heads as opposed to the Passiflora patients who feel everything in their hearts. The following story illustrates two people intuitively reaching for the medicine best suited to heal their anxiety.

Business partners John and Cynthia stopped by a local restaurant to decompress after leaving a difficult meeting during which they were informed that the group who had hired them had decided not to pay for work they had already completed. John had a more cerebral response than Susan. Although he was stressed and nervous he tried to analyze the situation intellectually. Susan, on the other hand, was hurt, tearful, and angry.

When the waiter came by to take their order, John instinctively ordered a beer (hops) while Susan ordered a cup of Passiflora tea.

Kava Kava (Piper methysticum) Piperaceae

Kava acts as an analgesic, anti-inflammatory, anti-fungal, and calming hypnotic sedative. Unlike other nervines, however, kava sharpens mental focus and increases concentration at the same time as it calms the nervous system. It is a wonderful addition to a musculoskeletal anti-spasmodic formula, where small amounts serve to potentize the entire formula. It may also be employed to reduce the discomfort and anxiety associated with interstitial cystitis. Lactones and kava lactones contained in the roots of kava are considered the important constituents responsible for the plant's ability to relax and sharpen the mind.

Traditionally a cold water extract is ritually prepared and the plant is ingested in conjunction with prayer. Kava Ceremonies are often performed before important meetings to enable participants to rise to a higher place within them selves before discussing important and controversial matters. Among the Samoans, and others, the first sip of Kava is always left as an offering to the Spirits.

Although large amounts of kava are consumed by natives of the Polynesian Islands, reports of hepatotoxicity, manifesting as elevated liver enzymes and the appearance of a dry, scaly, pigmented dermatitis, have largely been reported only in the west. The exact mechanism for toxicity has not been discovered, but it has been postulated that the use of benzene derivatives to extract and standardize kavalactones may be the culprit. In addition stem and leaf, discarded by natives, have in some cases been eagerly taken up by westerners due to the higher concentration of kavalactones in those parts of the plant. The native practice of not utilizing those plant parts for medicine suggests that stem and leaf may have toxic constituents not present in the roots. Cold water extractions ingested with prayerful intention might be the best way to use this plant, but kava has been safely utilized by many people over the years that it has been on the market. When symptoms of liver toxicity do occur they cease once the herb is discontinued. The suspected standardized extract is not necessary for full effect to occur with use of kava and may therefore easily be avoided. Like any standardized extract, the possibility of contamination with chemicals used for extraction of specific constituents may be significant. As kavalactones are not water soluble and are destroyed by heat, cold extractions can be made by squeezing infused herb through cheese cloth or other suitable material to extract the kavalactones.

I do not hesitate to use a tincture of kava in formulas for musculoskeletal spasm, and it is an excellent addition to any formula created for the cessation of smoking in the patient who has the will and determination to quit. I have also used it in formula with other nervines to help patients discontinue benzodiazepines. It can act as an analgesic agent in the treatment of fibromyalgia, where combines well with Actea/Cimicifuga racemosa and Piscidia.

When I want to nourish the nervous system for simple anxiety or insomnia however, I do not run to Kava except as a synergizer, as there are many other soothing and restorative herbs that are quite reliable for the job. More out of respect for its place as a Sacred Ceremonial Plant than from fear of potential toxicity, I prefer to use kava for specific indications, as a synergist in musculoskeletal formulas, as an analgesic, as an adjunct in the treatment of addiction, or as an ally to facilitate a deeper connection to the Divine and alleviate spiritual unrest.

Lavender (Lavendula angustifolia)

Lavender flowers contain bitter constituents that stimulate liver, gall bladder and digestive function. They are specifically indicated for bilious, toxic, or migraine headaches where they combine well with feverfew to treat acute headaches and prevent their recurrence. As a nervine, lavender acts to nourish and protect the nervous system from the toxins excreted as a result of the liver stimulating effects of the strong bitters in the feverfew. (See chapter on premenstrual headaches for more.)

In tincture, lavender combines well with other nervines for anxiety and nervousness, especially when toxemia and poor digestion contribute to nervous unrest.

Case

A 72 year old woman, whose insomnia was not responding to treatment with strong sedative herbs including valerian and passionflower, was advised to place some freshly dried lavender flowers into a clean cotton sock, tie off the end, and lay it near her face on retiring. She was also told to crush the flowers a bit each night without opening the sock, and take several deep breaths, inhaling the essential oils, before lying down to sleep with her makeshift lavender pillow. The results were spectacular. She went from experiencing little to no rest all night to sleeping like a baby.

This idea came to me after an article crossed my desk describing an incident in Great Britain where it was noted that the residents of a nursing home slept better when moved into a newly remodeled wing while elders in the old wing continued to experience varying degrees of the type of insomnia often experienced with increasing age. Because lavender has a folkloric reputation for being preferred by elders, the walls of the new wing had been papered with essential oil of lavender.

Lemon Balm (Melissa officinalis) Lamiaceae

The soft leaves of Melissa officinalis emit a sweet lemony scent that makes the plant a fine addition to a summer sun tea. Like other members of the mint family, the essential oils of lemon balm have carminative activity helpful for digestion.

Anti-viral properties make Melissa useful for the treatment of viral infections where it has gained popularity in recent years as a topical agent for acute flare-ups of herpes virus eruptions on skin and mucous membranes.[42] The addition of an internal formula of anti viral herbs will hasten healing in these cases far more effectively than a topical treatment used alone.

As an anti-spasmodic, Melissa's action is mild but supportive when used in formula with other nervines more specific for the treatment of spasm. Vasodilating actions contribute to a mild activity in lowering elevations in blood pressure.

As a nervine, lemon balm is effective, safe, and nontoxic, and may be used in children as well as adults. It is mildly antidepressant as well as calming for patients with anxiety. Antioxidants present in the plant contribute to give it anti-inflammatory activity.

Melissa's actions on thyroid metabolism make useful in the treatment of hyperthyroidism, where it combines well with Leonurus and Lycopus. Here Melissa acts by preventing the uptake of iodine for synthesis of T4 and conversion of T4 to active hormone T3 in peripheral tissues (primarily the liver). It also blocks binding of the pituitary hormone TSH to thyroid cell membranes,[43] another mechanism for preventing synthesis of thyroid hormone. In Graves' disease, Melissa will prevent the binding of thyroid autoimmune antibodies contributing to hyper function of the gland.[44]

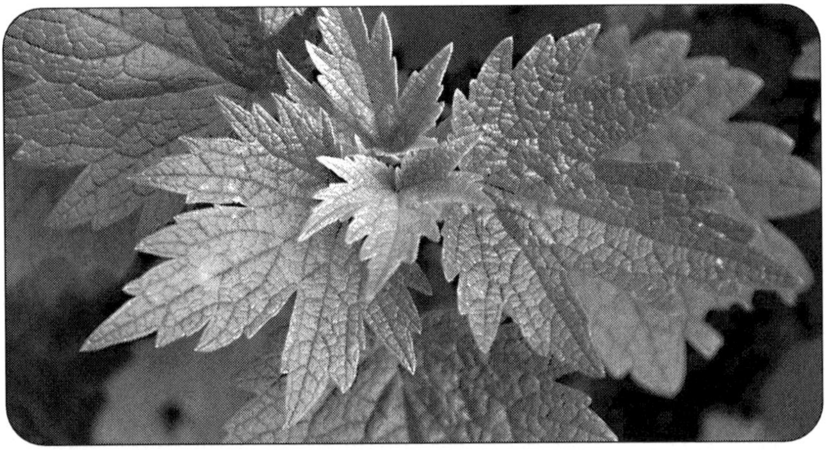

Motherwort *Photo courtesy of Tammi Miller*

Motherwort (Leonurus cardiaca) Labiatae

Another member of the mint family, motherwort is often combined with Melissa in the treatment of hyperthyroidism, where it acts to protect the heart and calm the cardiac plexus, both of which can become overstimulated by the increase in circulating thyroid hormone.

The species name "cardiaca" is given to the plant in recognition of its fine ability to correct functional heart palpitations that arise in the absence of organic cardiac disease and are usually associated with stress or anxiety.

Culpepper, a seventeenth century botanist and herbalist, suggests that Leonurus may have some anti-depressant powers. "There is no better herb to drive melancholy vapours from the heart, to strengthen it and make the mind cheerful, blithe and merry."

Early twentieth century herbalist, Maud Grieve, agrees when she writes in her the second volume of her book entitled "A Modern Herbal", "old writers tell us there is no better herb for gladdening and strengthening the heart..."

Motherwort has earned her common name from her ability to soothe the distraught nerves of overworked mothers and menopausal women. Unlike other members of the mint family, which are usually more soft and inviting, Leonurus presents as a bit tough and prickly, a fitting doctrine of signatures for encouraging women to honor their own prickliness and be assertive to get the space they need, before getting frazzled. It has been my experience that a few drops of tincture or a cup of the tea will enhance meditation practice when the focus of our intention is to deepen our connection to Divine Mother.

In menopause, motherwort is used for hot flashes, night sweats, and vaginal dryness as well as cardiac palpitations. It can also be used in younger women for the relief of symptoms associated with PMS, particularly when uterine cramping precedes the onset of menses. It may be helpful in bringing on delayed menses and is specific where pelvic achiness or lumbar discomfort are present, especially when accompanied by a bearing down sensation. It has also been employed for infertility, and postpartum depression associated with restlessness and anxiety.

Leonurus has also been used for neuralgia, neuritis, and as an aid in recovery from neurological conditions generally. It may be used for rheumatism, fever, tremors and nervous fatigue. The plant is somewhat astringent and diaphoretic.

A tea may be prepared by infusing 1 teaspoon of dried leaves into a cup of water. A 1:1 tincture may be dosed at 10-40 drops and dispensed 2-4 times per day.

For cardiac palpitations Leonurus combines well with Crataegus spp. (hawthorne) where equal parts of the two herbs can be mixed in the tincture and dosed at 60 drops three times per day. It rarely fails in the treatment of functional heart palpitations when constitutional issues are also addressed.

Leonurus acts as a pelvic decongestant and emmenogogue when menses are sluggish in starting or delayed in onset. As a uterine tonic and anti-spasmodic nervine, it is useful for treating menstrual or premenstrual cramps that occur in an attempt to get delayed or sluggish menstrual flow moving. It may also act as an oxytocic agent. Leonurus can be of aid in alleviating premenstrual tension, water retention, and menopausal symptoms.

Constituents include flavonoids, glycosides, and several alkaloids. The leaves are used for medicine.

Oats (Avena sativa) Poaceae

Milky oat seeds contain protein and are high in minerals, including silica, calcium, magnesium, zinc and iron, making them a highly nutritive plant. They also contain saponins, flavonoids, and alkaloids. The seeds are trophorestorative to nervous tissue, and should therefore be considered part of a total protocol for the treatment of neurological conditions. Boericke[45] suggests the use of oats for treating patients with addictions. Used alone I have not seen much effect in these situations, but Avena should certainly not be underestimated as an adjunctive herb in these cases.

Both milky oat seed and the grain we use as food have a calming influence and both can be dosed freely.

Skullcap (Scutellaria lateriflora) Lamiaceae

Eclectic practitioners[46] used Scutellaria specifically for musculoskeletal spasm, tremors and twitching. The presence of several anti-inflammatory, anti-oxidant flavonoids contributes to reduce toxemia as a potential etiology for musculoskeletal irritability, emotional anxiety, agitation and restlessness.

Amelioration of muscle spasm extends to the heart muscle where the plant has been found useful in alleviating functional heart palpitations. Although Leonurus, which has proven so trustworthy in treating functional heart palpitations, has become my personal preference in these cases, Scutellaria should also be considered, especially if symptoms of cardiac irregularity are accompanied by spasm and twitching elsewhere in the body. The plant should also be considered as an adjunct in the treatment of hypertension.

Scutellaria increases circulation to the cerebral cortex and is considered to be trophorestorative to the nervous system, making it a strong consideration for use in neurological conditions, particularly when an injury or insult to the nervous system manifests in symptoms of nervous agitation, difficulty concentrating, anxiety, and insomnia. Recent research with animals suggests Scutellaria may be effective in the treatment of seizures.[47]

Bitter principles present in the plant aid in improving digestive function.

Sedative properties make skullcap useful for the treatment of insomnia due to excessive worry and nervous agitation.

Constituents include ten flavonoids and two glycosides.[48]

St. John's Wort (Hypericum perforatum) Hypericaceae

St. John's Wort received a lot of press some years ago as an anti-depressant. Shortly thereafter, a few poorly done studies revealed that it was not active as an anti-depressant. One of the studies was done with a severely depressed population, for whom Hypericum would not be expected to work in any case.

The truth is that St. John's wort often works very well in mild to moderate depression and is specific for seasonal affective disorder. While it may prove helpful as an adjunct for more serious depression, it is not specifically indicated for that condition, except perhaps as a supportive herb.

In addition to being an anti-depressant, calming nervine, St. John's Wort also possesses anti-viral properties. It may be used internally and externally for herpes infections on skin and mucous membranes.[49] One herbalist told me she had used an oil of Hypericum topically with success in a case of herpes zoster (shingles). Because the herpes viruses reside in nerve roots and herpes zoster in particular causes its eruption along a dermatomal nerve pathway, Hypericum, which is trophorestorative to nerve tissue as well as anti-viral, is well indicated for herpes infections. When symptoms confirm, homeopathic Rhus tox can also be effective for treating the painful eruptions of herpes zoster, especially when used in conjunction with anti-viral herbs taken internally and applied topically. Aggressive dosing of anti-viral herb should be employed for acute cases of herpes outbreaks. Flavonoids add anti-inflammatory, anti-oxidant and hepato-protective activities.

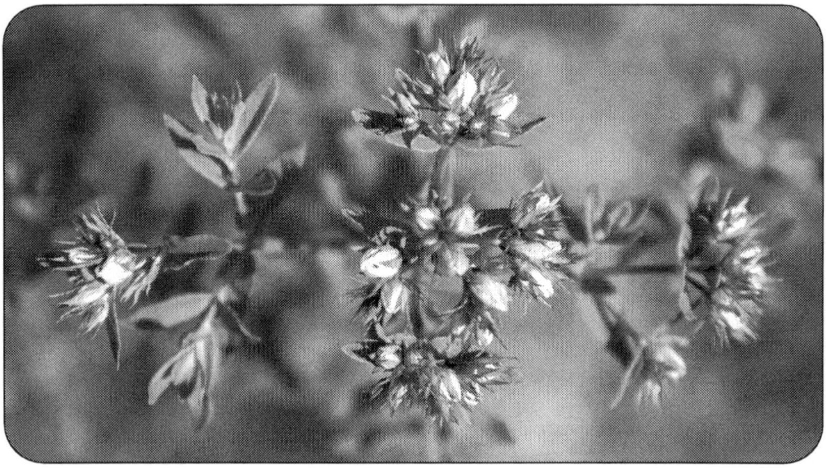

St. John's Wort, spring buds *Photo courtesy of Tammi Miller*

St. John's Wort has spiritually protective qualities that have a special affinity for the reproductive tract. Recognizing that women are more sensitive and open during menses, women in traditional cultures in Europe painted their labias with an oil of Hypericum for protection during moontime. I have had numerous experiences in clinic using the oil topically for protection from unsolicited, inappropriate sexual advances, when the woman who was the object of the predatory stalking was experiencing physical symptoms of restless agitation in the pelvic area. One application of a few drops of the oil of Hypericum and the restless agitation will, more often than not, completely disappear.

Hypericum has a strong mythological connection to the sun and is named for the pre-Olympian Greek God of the sun, Hyperion. Long associated with magic, the yellow flowers turn a deep blood red when placed into menstruum for medicine making, reminding us of the life giving energy of the sun.

Formula for Acute Herpes Virus Outbreaks

Melissa officinalis	1 - 2 drams or 5 10 ml.
Hypericum perforatum	1 dram or 5 ml.
Glycerrhiza glabra	1 dram or 5 ml.
Lomatium dissectum	2 drams or 10 ml.
Ligusticum porteri	1 - 2 drams or 5 - 10 ml.
Echinacea	1 dram or 5 ml.

The total amount of all the herbs mixed together should equal 8 drams per ounce or 30 ml. per ounce.

The use of several herbs in the formula allows for frequent dosing which is often preferable in acute illnesses or flare-ups of chronic conditions. This particular formula may be given 30 - 60 drops every two hours for 48 hours while the patient is awake, then reduced to every 4 hours for several more days, or as long as is needed. For prevention of acute eruptions, the formula may be given at doses of 30 - 60 drops 3 - 4 times per day.

Glycerrhiza, Melissa, and Hypericum may all be used for the topical treatment of herpes infections. For optimal healing to occur, it is vital to also dose the patient with an oral regimen of immune-supportive, anti-viral herbs, as illustrated in the formula above. Treating the skin alone neglects internal needs for immune enhancement and nerve healing.

Passionflower
(Passiflora incarnata) Passifloraceae

Passiflora is a gentle but effective sedative for insomnia due to overwork, overexcitement, mental congestion, worry, shock, or heartache. It is especially useful for insomnia related to prolonged illness, debility with nervousness from inactivity, and for insomnia after an acute illness with fever. It may be mixed in formula with other herbs if higher doses are required to induce sleep.

Passiflora is well indicated for spasmodic conditions, where it may be used alone or in combination with other herbs. It has been used as a helpful adjunct in quieting the spasm of whooping cough or spasmodic asthma. It can also be helpful in warding off migraine if given at the first sign of the aura that often accompanies migraines. Similarly, it is a medicine to consider for tension headache or musculo-skeletal tension and spasm in general. Passiflora's anti-spasmodic actions extend to the smooth muscles of blood vessels where it can aid in lowering elevated blood pressure. Flavonoids add anti-inflammatory properties.

Although I find Leonurus to be our most reliable medicine for the treatment of functional heart palpitations, Passiflora is also indicated for palpitations, especially if due to lack of sleep or general anxiety and tension.

Passiflora is safe for infants to old folks, although milder, less sedating herbs such as California poppy, lemon balm, catnip, or chamomile often work well for the little ones.

For the treatment of insomnia, a formula of the above mentioned herbs or any one used as a simple can be given in tincture at a dose of 60 drops 1 -2 hours before retiring, followed by a second dose right at bedtime. Adrenal adaptogens and/or smaller doses of the sedative nervine formula should be given 2 - 3 times during the day to support adrenal function and calm and soothe the nervous system throughout the day.

Constituents include the alkaloid harmoline, a cyanide glycoside gynocardin, flavonoids, maltol and harmon.

Jamaican Dogwood
(Piscidia erythina, P. piscipula) Fabaceae

Piscidia is a dose sensitive plant with potential for toxicity and should therefore be used with caution. The plant is reported to be an effective analgesic without the problems of constipation that accompany the use of opiates. When used in proper doses it is generally without side effects.

Piscidia's analgesic activities include significant anti-spasmodic actions. It is highly efficacious for musculoskeletal spasm, intestinal, gall bladder, or renal colic, dysmenorrhea, and spasmodic coughs, including pertussis (whooping cough).

Anti-inflammatory activity exhibited by Piscidia is due at least in part to the presence of flavonoids. It has been helpful for alleviating the pain of fibromyalgia, migraine headache, arthritis, and pelvic pain. As a sedative nervine it is effective for insomnia and anxiety due to cerebral congestion, worry, overexcitement, and over exhaustion.

Piscidia is said to be specific for neuralgia and may be considered for the pain of herpes zoster or facial neuralgia.

Symptoms of toxicity from overdose include decreased sensation, muscular laxity, incoordination, increased salivation, diaphoresis, increased then decreased pupil size, drowsiness, diminished reflexes, bradycardia (lowered heart rate), increased then decreased blood pressure, convulsions, respiratory paralysis, general paralysis and finally, death.

The roots are used in medicine. A 1:5 tincture may be dosed at 5 - 30 drops, up to 3 times per day.

Valerian (Valeriana spp.) Valerianaceae

The gentle but effective passion flower acts like a loving grandmother who softly rocks us to sleep, while the energy of valerian seems more masculine and assertive in its actions. Valerian is certainly an effective sedative hypnotic, and although the occasional patient will have an idiosyncratic response and become agitated by the herb, I have actually only seen this on a few occasions.

For insomnia, dosing of 60 drops either as a simple or in combination with other nervines or sedative herbs should be taken one to two hours before retiring, with another dose taken at bedtime. Doses can be repeated as needed throughout the night. If too much valerian is taken, the patient will wake with a heavy, hung over feeling in the morning in which case the dose should be reduced. Other sedative herbs, such as Passiflora are less likely to have this effect.

Valerian is an effective antispasmodic in the musculoskeletal system as well as in the treatment of dysmenorrhea. Hypotensive properties may be of help for patients struggling with high blood pressure. The plant is also reputed to have anti-convulsant activity.

The roots are used in medicine, and although the plant may be dispensed as a tea, the essential oils do not emit a very pleasant aroma, so tincture or capsules are more often employed.

Constituents include volatile oils, sesquiterpenes, a few amino acids, alkaloids, and valpotriates.

Vervain (Verbena offficinalis, V. hastata) Verbenaceae

Vervain is specifically indicated for patients whose nerves are frayed and strained to the last degree. The irritability and edginess that the patient experiences might be likened to the sort of feeling that occurs if someone nearby is continually scraping their fingernails down a chalkboard. This herb also helps in easing the depression and inner torment that often accompanies symptoms of nervous irritability. In any of these cases the addition of even a small amount of vervain to a formula of nervines helps the whole prescription work more effectively.

Years ago, when I was a budding herbalist and still ignorant about vervain's astringent and drying effects, I took vervain for some vague nervous symptoms while concurrently experiencing some mild coryza, or cold symptoms. The drying effect of the herb led to a suppression of the discharge that resulted in sinus pressure and pain where previously there had only been a mild, clear nasal discharge. Although it eased my nervous unrest, it was clearly not the appropriate herb in that moment.

Bitter principles in the herb aid digestive function and the plant is an effective alterative. Despite its drying properties, it has emmenogogue and galactogogue properties and has been used to ease the tension of menopause. Folklore gives it a reputation as an aphrodisiac.

Writer John Lust (The Herb Book) suggests that the tincture may be dosed at 20 to 40 drops as needed. Powdered herb can be dispensed 1/4 to 1/2 teaspoon three times per day while tea should ideally be prepared as a cold extract, using one tablespoon per cup of water and allowing the plant to infuse for several hours before drinking. One cup of tea per day is his recommended dose and I might suggest drinking that one cup over the course of the day or taking 1/3 of the cup three times per day with meals in order to take better advantage of the digestive bitters contained in the herb.

I have personally found that this herb works well in small doses of only 3 - 5 drops 3 - 4 times per day. It is an excellent synergist when added in small doses to a formula of nervines.

European vervain (Verbena officinalis) was used by the Druids for divination, ritual cleansing, and spiritual protection. Some Native American people used the American species (Verbena hastata) to drive away undesirable spirits.

Kali Phosphoricum

A few pellets of a 6X or 12X potency of this cell salt may be taken four times per day to calm and heal an overwrought nervous system. Alternatively, one or two pellets can be placed right into a tincture of nervines to potentize the formula. The tincture may still be given as often as needed.

Cell salts, such as this one, are low dose homeopathic medicines that have an affinity for specific tissues, where they act to stimulate healing. The remedies are readily available in most health food stores and generally come in 6X or 12 X potencies. Average dosing for most cell salts is a few pellets 4 times daily. Although more frequent dosing may sometimes be employed, it is usually not necessary. These remedies can be given along with constitutional homeopathics without interference in most cases.

Dosing Strategies

Nervines can be dosed several times a day either in formula or as simples. When patients present with really significant symptoms of nervous tension, however, a combination of several herbs in formula allows for higher and more frequent dosing.

A tincture combining 6 - 8 herbs can be administered every 1 - 2 hours for as long as is needed, reducing to every 4 hours after symptoms begin to ease. This strategy is particularly useful for treating patients struggling to ward off a psychotic episode or who feel so stressed they fear they may end up breaking down.

Another dosage strategy is to use a tea of nervine herbs, infusing 4 tablespoons of the herbal blend into a quart of water. The patient is then instructed to sip the tea throughout the day. It has been my experience that this class of herbs does best when taken in this way. Alternatively a tincture can be dispensed with instructions to place 1 - 2 teaspoons into a quart water bottle to be sipped throughout the day.

Flower essences, when indicated, can be added right into tincture bottles for easy dispensing.

Other Considerations

Needless to say there are dozens of other therapies that can be helpful in mitigating symptoms of insomnia and nervous tension. Space does not allow us to cover all possibilities, but a few other helpful hints are listed below. Attention to blood sugar imbalances and other constitutional problems are essential for optimal healing.

Neutral Bath

This simple therapy was commonly utilized in psychiatric institutions before the introduction of psychoactive pharmaceuticals. An acquaintance who worked as a nurse on a psychiatric unit once shared a case with me confirming the traditional use of the neutral bath. A pregnant woman who was forcibly brought to the hospital due to a highly agitated and manic state was placed in four point restraints to keep her from hurting herself or others. Because the woman was pregnant, the usual drugs could not be employed to settle her down. The nurse insisted that the patient be released to her custody for a badly needed bath. She reported that the patient instinctively drew a bath of completely neutral temperature, which served to pull her out of her agitated state.

To calm overwrought nerves, simply prepare a bath that is completely neutral in temperature, feeling neither warm nor cool to the bather. Although the average temperature to achieve the desired sedative effect runs from 93 - 97 degrees, it is not necessary to measure the temperature of the water, as the patient's subjective sensation of a neutral temperature is adequate. Twenty minutes in the bath is usually long enough to induce relaxation.

Warming Socks

This treatment helps alleviate insomnia by drawing congestion from the head. While it is commonly used when congestion is due to respiratory issues or fluid retention, it is also effective for mental congestion. The patient should be warm before the treatment is started and if the feet are cold they should be warmed in hot water before proceeding.

A pair of cotton socks is soaked in very cold water and wrung out thoroughly. These socks are placed on the feet, and then covered by another pair of socks, made of material that will not absorb the water, such as wool or synthetic fleece. The patient goes to bed for the night with the two pairs of socks on the feet, and by morning the cotton socks will be dry.

Although this treatment sounds uncomfortable, it is usually only a matter of minutes before the body warms up the wet socks and the uncomfortable sensation disappears.

Chapter 5
The Art of Herbal Formulating

WHEN WE LOOK OUT INTO NATURE, we can see that plants often grow very close together, easily sharing space with other plants. Branches from neighboring trees gently brush one another in the wind. Roots cross over each other underground, and some plants, like Pedicularis, pull constituents from surrounding plants. Certainly there are exceptions. The desert chaparral (Larrea tridentate), for example, puts out constituents that deter the growth of other plant life, even its own offspring. All in all, though, plants seem to thrive in a community setting. I often think they could teach us humans a thing or two about how we might better get along with each other!

It is no surprise then that herbs are commonly prescribed as formulas, allowing plants to blend their healing properties in a synergistic way that often results in more than the sum of the parts.

Tips for the Creation of Herbal Formulas

There are no hard and fast rules for formulating, but the following ideas may offer a few tips for organizing your thoughts so you can then organize your herbs!

What is the patient's chief complaint and how crucial is it to specifically address that complaint in the formula?

Which organs or organ systems are involved and which of these must be addressed in order to obtain the greatest healing in an efficient and gentle manner? In other words which organ(s) should be prioritized and which organ(s) should be nourished or toned to support the primary organ being treated?

For example, a patient with arthritis may report with a chief complaint of joint pain. While a simple prescription of Harpagophytum procumbens (devil's claw), an herb specific for joint pain, will likely address that chief complaint, the patient will usually fare much better if we add herbs that support adrenal function and aid in elimination of toxins that are likely contributing to joint pain and inflammation. Such a formula might include other anti-inflammatory herbs, such as Salix or Actea/Cimicifuga, to enhance the action of the Harpagophytum and reduce the need to rely on a plant that must be imported from Africa. Because the the joints are known to drain through the kidney channel, juniper or chimaphila might be added to support the kidneys in eliminating toxins.

How much do mental, emotional, and spiritual issues play into the picture? Is a mental block or a fixed idea aggravating or causing symptoms? Is the illness causing emotional distress or is emotional stress contributing to symptoms? Will a good adrenal formula suffice or do we need to be more specific? We might choose Aralia to help an emotionally closed patient begin to trust and open the heart, allowing a let a little of the world in again. Perhaps Rhodiola or Crataegus should be added to help alleviate grief, or a nervine and/or adaptogen for general nervousness and fear.

Is the patient warm, chilly, thirsty, dry, moist, or damp? A chilly patient will do best with ginger in a digestive formula, while the warmer patient might prefer the more cooling peppermint.

In what form do we want to dispense our medicine? Shall we use tincture, tea, powder, capsule, or solid extract, or can we simply incorporate the herb into the diet? We may want to dispense a tea to emphasize fluid intake. Patients with respiratory or urinary tract infections may take our advice to drink more fluids if we medicate their water. Sometimes a tea can help a patient create a ritual for self care and quiet time, where another patient, overburdened by fatigue and too many responsibilities may be vexed by having one more thing to do.

If we are using herbs to treat osteoporosis or to facilitate optimal healing of a recent fracture, a tincture, while convenient and easy, will not necessarily serve the purpose, as desired mineral constituents will not extract well into alcohol. A vinegar extract of mineral rich herbs may be preferable, particularly as vinegar not only extracts minerals from the plant, but also adds acid for enhanced uptake of minerals in the digestive tract. Teas and inclusion of whole or powdered herbs in food will also deliver minerals better than tincture.

Is it practical for the patient to make tea or mix powders into food? Does fatigue, emotional stress, or overwork simply burden our patient further if we ask them to mix a powder into food or make a tea? How do the herbs in our formula taste? Strong tasting plants like feverfew, very bitter and unpleasant in taste, may be better prescribed in capsule or tincture than as a tea.

Can we individualize our formula if we use capsules? Will individualization of the formula enhance results for this patient or do we have a premixed formula on the shelf that will work just fine?

What do we have easily available, either in our offices or in the surrounding community? How do financial considerations play in?

Tinctures have become a common route of administration for herbs, offering longer shelf life, more opportunity to individualize formulas, and more ease of administration for patients, but there are other considerations that may contraindicate the use of alcohol besides the desire to deliver a mineral rich formula. Is the patient alcoholic and fearful of using tinctures? Does serious liver disease contraindicate the use of alcohol? Some important plant constituents like resins in Grindelia or Eriodictyon are important for their expectorant actions in treating cough. Resins extract better in alcohol than water, making tincture more appealing. Demulcent herbs such as Althea do best when given as a cold water infusion. Recent personal experience with a glycerite extraction of bilberry suggests that glycerine extracts may enhance peripheral vasodilatory actions when selecting bilberry. A tannin rich herb combined in formula with an herb high in alkaloids may cause toxic alkaloids to precipitate out and settle in the bottom of the tincture bottle, potentially creating problems for toxic dosing as the bottle nears empty.

Can we do all we want with one formula or will we dilute the strength of our formula by trying to do too much? Will the patient take more than one formula? For example, it may be more efficacious to dose liver stimulating herbs separately, increasing or decreasing doses as tolerated, while leaving other herbs as originally prescribed. Similarly, nervines or anti-spasmodic formulas may do best as a separate formula to allow for flexibility in dosing as needed.

How sensitive is the patient? Do we need to limit the number of herbs we place into the formula so we can more easily identify which herb is the culprit if a sensitivity issue arises?

A common method that herbalists use when teaching principles of formulation is to think of each formula as containing a lead herb or herbs, supporting herbs, a driver and possibly a synergist.

The lead herb is the plant that we expect to carry out the main actions needed. For example in an acutely infected skin wound our lead herb for an internal formula might be Echinacea. It stimulates immune function, has been shown to be anti-bacterial against staphylococcus, and streptococcus, and aids the body in dealing with underlying issues of toxemia.

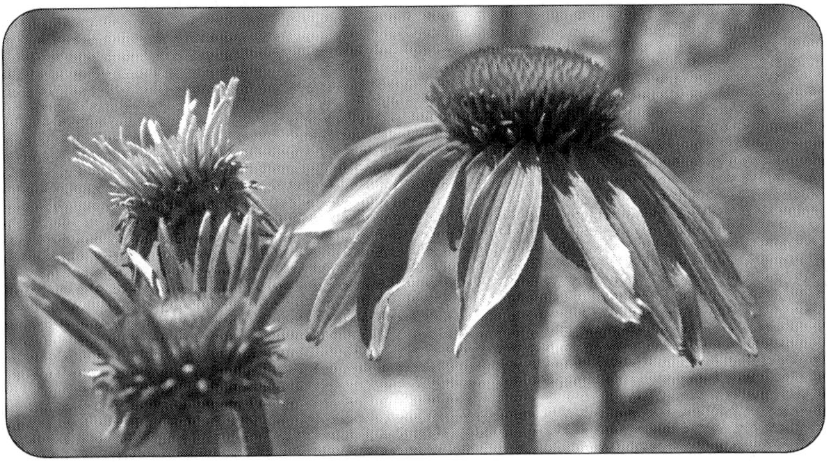

Echinacea *Photo courtesy of Tammi Miller*

Supporting herbs are added into a formula to enhance the actions of the lead herb. They may act by adding to the actions of the lead herb, nourishing the other organs critical to the process, or by covering the case with another related but important action. So for the infected wound we might add Myrrh to support the immune enhancing properties of the Echinacea.

Drivers are plants that take the formula to the designated site, where "it's all happening.'" They may be herbs that stimulate circulation or target a specific organ or part of the body. In the case of our infected wound, cayenne or ginger might be added as warming circulatory stimulants. In a case of ovarian cysts, Caulophyllum, with its specificity to pelvic organs and to ovaries in particular, will act as both a lead herb and driver.

The synergist is a plant that combines its actions with the other herbs to make the whole formula more effective. Strong, potentially toxic plants and essential oils are often used as synergists. As a lymphatic, immune herb, and blood cleanser, small doses of Baptisia combine well with Echinacea as a synergist in the case of the infected wound.

If, on the other hand, we are treating a case of premenstrual breast tenderness, we might choose Ceanothus spp. as our lead herb. Ceanothus is specific for premenstrual breast tenderness, but also adds supporting action by enhancing liver function and decreasing inflammation and toxicity. A driver effect is present due to the plant's affinity for breast and lymphatic tissue. Here we see that one herb covers a number of actions. In this case, Ceanothus may be the only herb needed.

In another situation, a woman comes in with dysmenorrhea (painful cramping with menses). In this case uterine tonics such as Angelica sinensis, Viburnum opulus, Actea (Cimicifuga) racemosa, or Rubus spp. will improve tone to the uterine muscle when given all month long. If we select Angelica as our lead herb in this case, we would not necessarily need a driver as the lead herb already has activity as a pelvic decongestant with specificity to the uterine muscle.

More than one uterine tonic may be included in a formula for complimentary and synergistic actions. Perhaps our patient has a scanty flow of blood (Angelica sinensis) and tends towards depression or has a history of sexual abuse. (Cimicifuga racemosa). Then we would want to include both herbs in the formula. If premenstrual breast tenderness is also a symptom, Ceanothus could be added as a supportive pelvic decongestant that addresses another symptom.

Supportive herbs may also include flower essences, if emotional issues are creating concern.

Flower essences are similar to homeopathic medicines in the sense that they are dilutions and work as vibrational medicine, affecting the emotional, spiritual, and mental state of the patient. The essences are made by infusing fresh, good quality flowers in a bowl of water set in the sun for a period of four hours. They are then preserved by the addition of alcohol. Further dilution allows the essences to be dispensed in dropper bottles for oral administration. Different essences may be mixed into one bottle for ease of dosing, if more than one essence seems indicated.

Chapter 6 *Musculoskeletal System*

Spasm and Inflammation

Medicinal plants quite wisely recognize that tense or spasmodic muscles are often accompanied by mental or emotional stress. Not coincidentally, the group of herbs that addresses spasm in the musculoskeletal system is composed largely of the nervines that calm and soothe the nervous system.

When creating a formula for musculoskeletal spasm, it may be optimal to include anti-inflammatory herbs as well as anti-spasmodics, as there is often some level of inflammation whenever spasm is present. Some herbs, such as Actea/Cimicifuga racemosa, Pedicularis spp., and Viburnum opulus, are both anti-spasmodic and anti-inflammatory. In contrast, Salix spp. is not anti-spasmodic but will aid in alleviating inflammation. Not all anti-spasmodic herbs are appropriate for skeletal muscle spasm. Chamomile, for example, is specific for spasm and inflammation in the digestive tract, while mullein is anti-spasmodic and demulcent in the intestines and respiratory tract.

The formula that follows provides a template for formulas that have been highly effective in clinic. Variations in the formula will depend on individual patient needs and availability of herbs. For example, the addition of Passiflora may be desirable if emotional heartache contributes to spasm. Valerian may be contraindicated for the odd patient who reacts to the herb by becoming more agitated. Concomitant depression, hormonal imbalances, or a tendency to menstrual cramps may favor the addition of Cimicifuga. The practitioner may want to place more emphasis on herbs that modulate inflammation, such as Cimicifuga, Viburnum and Pedicularis, if inflammation is complicating spasm more than in another case. Finally, the practical reality may be that the formula will be modified according to what is available at the moment.

Vigorous, frequent dosing in the first 48 hours is essential to break through the wall of spasm. Frequency of administration can then be decreased except in the most severe cases. Because these herbs act to reduce muscle spasm and inflammation, a formula of this group of herbs, administered in conjunction with spinal manipulation, helps the correction to hold better when frequent dosing is employed.

Actea/Cimicifuga racemosa	1 dram
Viburnum opulus	1 dram
Piper methysticum	1 dram
Pedicularis spp	2 drams
Valeriana officinalis and/or Passiflora	1 dram
Scutellaria lateriflora	1 dram
Eschscholzia californica	1 dram

Administer 60 drops every 2 hours while awake for the first 2 days, then decrease to every 4 hours for 2 days, continuing to taper off in frequency as symptoms improve. The inclusion of several herbs in the formula allows for higher doses to be given frequently without danger of overdosing any one herb. The formula may be given long term at 30 to 60 drops 3 - 6 times daily when chronic conditions warrant continued usage.

The herb Pedicularis spp. often proves useful as a simple in allaying muscle tension and inflammation. Doses of 60 drops given 5 - 6 times a day for the first two days are usually just as effective at alleviating acute spasm as the more frequent dosing of the formula. The dose may then be tapered as symptoms indicate.

Many products available on the market will include magnesium in their formulations to allay spasm. Magnesium can be taken in doses of 50 to 100 milligrams every 2 hours for 24 hours then dropped to every 4 hours for the next day or two. Excessive magnesium can lead to diarrhea and gas, in which case dosage should be decreased.

Bromelain, an enzyme extracted from pineapple, is a very effective anti-inflammatory agent. It is readily available on the market and can be dosed at 500 to 1000 mg 3 - 4 times per day or more often as needed. I am unaware of any negative effects and have taken as much as 500 milligrams every 2 hours myself. It combines well with turmeric for inflammation, where the two agents taken together seem to work better than either one alone. Encapsulated formulas containing both turmeric and bromelain can be found in some health food stores.

Belladonna (Atropa belladonna) Solanaceae

Belladonna is generally only available to licensed health care practitioners as it is a highly toxic plant that must be dosed conservatively. This plant cuts through spasm when nothing else makes a dent. It should be included with other anti-spasmodic herbs as a synergist to make the entire formula more effective.

Thirty (30) drops of the 1:10 tincture made from dried herb are placed into a 4 ounce bottle with a teaspoon or two of alcohol added as a preservative. The bottle is then filled with water sufficient to make a total volume of 4 ounces.

Doses of 1 teaspoon every 2 hours of this diluted mix are usually adequate, although the herb can be taken every hour. Maximum dose for a 130 - 150 pound adult is 24 teaspoons in 24 hours. In severe cases, teaspoon doses can be repeated every 15 minutes for 3 - 4 doses then dropped back to every one to two hours.

Overdose symptoms of Belladonna include dry mouth, dilated pupils, staggering, unsteady gait, increased thirst, flushed face, tachycardia, hypertension, and delirium. If overdose is significant convulsions, stupor and death may result.

Black Cohosh (Actea /Cimicfuga racemosa) Ranunculaceae

Although commonly thought of as a women's herb, black cohosh is highly effective as an anti-spasmodic and anti-inflammatory for musculoskeletal conditions in men or women. Ferulic acid and salicylic acid contained in the plant are thought to be responsible for its inflammatory actions.

Although Actea is specifically indicated for deep dark depression as well as anxiety, the depression does not need to be present to prescribe this plant.

Overdosing causes a dull frontal headache, which can proceed to hypotension and collapse if continued for very long.

Lobelia (Lobelia inflata) Lobeliaceae

Frequently employed internally for the treatment of asthma and other spasmodic conditions of the respiratory tract, lobelia can also be very effective as a topical agent in alleviating muscle spasm. I have witnessed remarkable results using topical applications of tincture, with reduction of spasm occurring almost instantly. Although it may not always be that dramatic in its action, such experiences should encourage its use as a topical agent. Wetted poultices of powdered or infused herb laid on the area of spasm may also prove efficacious.

When used internally, doses should be kept to no more than 60 drops in a 24 hour period, dispensed in divided doses. (1:2 strength) The actual toxicity of lobelia is disputed, but it is a powerful emetic and is sometimes used as such. Chances are that the vomiting produced by injudicious dosing would make ingestion of a truly toxic dose rather difficult.

Cramp Bark
(Viburnum opulus) Caprifoliaceae

This plant can be helpful in alleviating spasm and inflammation of the uterus, bronchial tree, and gastro-intestinal tract as well as skeletal muscle. The plant's astringency makes it especially valuable in treating menstrual cramps with excessive bleeding.

A close relative, Viburnum prunifolius, has also been used for alleviating spasm, but is generally considered to be less potent as an anti-spasmodic agent.

Both Viburnums are contraindicated in patients taking blood thinning medications.

Radiating Nerve Pain

Because radicular (radiating nerve) pain is usually accompanied by muscle spasm, the following therapies should be used in addition to herbs outlined above.

Homeopathic Agaricus, derived from the mushroom of the same name, (Agaricus muscarius) is highly effective at alleviating most cases of radicular pain. I have used it with great success, in conjunction with good physical medicine therapies, for patients who suffer from nerve impingement from various causes. It is also effective at reducing the muscle spasm caused or aggravated by nerve impingement. The remedy should be dosed at a potency of 30 C administered 4 times daily. Although other practitioners report using higher potencies with good effect the 30C has been most effective in my practice.

One patient, who was given 30C Agaricus four times daily for symptoms of severe cervical disc herniation, did remarkably well on all levels. The remedy ended up having deep acting constitutional affects for her, strengthening her mentally and emotionally, and healing hormonal imbalances, as well as her cervical disc herniations. When the 30C potency was increased to a 200C, the remedy stopped having the desired effects until we returned to the 30C.

A diabetic patient, who was given the remedy in one ounce of water instead of the usual sugar pellets, discovered that topical application was also effective in relieving flare ups of pain.

This remedy has proven highly reliable in relieving radicular pain in many cases in clinic and should also be considered for the paresthesias associated with nerve impingement. When Agaricus does not work, homeopathic Hypericum can be considered, prescribing the dose according to the severity of symptoms, a 30C frequently for more low grade chronic complaints, and a higher potency for more severe or acute flare ups of nerve pain.

Injections of 1000 micrograms of Vitamin B 12 given intra-muscularly may be added if symptoms persist. I often start by having patients do injections 3 times a week to start, tapering as symptoms improve.

Although it may not be necessary to use them in every case, herbs such as Centella asiatica (Gotu Kola), Hypericum Perforatum (St. John's Wort), and Avena sativa (Milky Oat Seed) are trophorestorative to the nervous system and should also be considered when radicular pain is present, to help repair irritated nerves.

Successful treatment of chronic musculoskeletal complaints can only be accomplished when we remember to treat the entire patient and not just the lesional symptoms or chief complaint. Inflammation will be unlikely to resolve if adrenal function is marginal. Spasm can be caused or aggravated by poor digestion, poor dietary habits, lack of sleep, liver congestion and toxemia, or chronic infection. Skeletal fixations must also be addressed in these cases.

Case

The following story was contributed by another naturopath who started out as one of my students.

"Five years ago when I was mentoring with you in Southern Oregon you invited me to bring my dog Butch into the office to be with us for the day. Due to chronic sciatica, he had difficulty mounting the few steps that led into the office, so you prescribed Agaricus 30 C and he improved remarkably.

Five years later, at fifteen, Butch is blind, deaf, and incontinent, but still eating and eager for hikes, until recently. Although he does not appear to be in any pain, his back legs have been failing. For the last few days, we have watched him try endlessly to stand, until finally he just gives up in exhaustion and has even stopped eating. We decided the time had come to let him go and I made an appointment with a local homeopathic veterinarian to have him euthanized the next day.

Shortly after calling the vet, I was returning some homeopathics to a shelf in my office, and saw the bottle of Agaricus I had made for him six years earlier. I remembered how we had used it for his back legs previously and decided to bring it home. I gave him a dose of the remedy just before bedtime. When the vet arrived in the morning, Butch leapt to his feet, sauntered across the slippery hardwood floor with grace, ate the entire contents of his food bowl, and for the first time in a year, shook his collar to communicate he wanted to go outside, and walked outside to poop!!

He has been fine for over a week now.

WooHoo Homeopathy! And thank YOU Dr. Frances."

Chapter 7

Digestive Function

THE DISCUSSION THAT FOLLOWS highlights a few simple treatment guidelines for selected conditions of the gastrointestinal tract and is not meant to be all inclusive.

ENHANCING DIGESTIVE FUNCTION

Proper nutrition is fundamental to any attempt to heal or maintain health. As discussed earlier, a healthy diet includes adequate protein, appropriate types and amounts of fats and carbohydrates, an abundance of fresh fruits and vegetables, and sufficient quantities of good quality water.

Tap water is generally not optimal as it contains a variety of chemicals used in the purification process to eradicate pathological bacteria. Filtered or clean spring water are options that many people are turning to in an attempt to avoid these toxic chemicals. It is also best to avoid plastic containers wherever possible, as plastic can leak endocrine disrupting chemicals into otherwise good quality water.

More and more people are experiencing difficulty maintaining optimal health on a carbohydrate rich diet, even when ingested carbs come from whole foods, such as brown rice or whole wheat. Grains seem to be poorly tolerated by many patients. Part of this shift is thought to be due to genetic alteration of many of the grains we eat.

Although these modifications may seem minor to some, the detrimental effects on health are significant. In addition, endocrine disrupting chemicals have become ubiquitous in the environment and are contributing to deterioration in liver and endocrine function, organ systems that are critical for healthy carbohydrate metabolism.[50]

For these reasons, many people are finding a need for increased protein consumption to keep blood sugars levels steady, and to provide the liver with the food it needs to breakdown toxins and bind them to lipo-proteins for transport to organs of elimination.

Good quality proteins include nuts, seeds, nut butters, raw unpasteurized organic milk, yogurt, and cheeses, eggs, and a wide variety of organic meats. Fish should be wild, not farmed, as farmed fish are often fed substances that change the beneficial fats found in fish to harmful fats. Red meat has gotten a bad reputation, but in fact some people will do better with red meat than chicken or turkey, as excessive amounts of poultry and eggs can place stress on the function of the gall bladder in susceptible individuals. It is something of an oddity that western medicine recommends poultry over red meat for lowering cholesterol, as the gall bladder is the only way that the liver eliminates excess cholesterol. Red meat should be organically raised and come from grass fed animals.

Care must be taken with ingestion of fish, as the oceans have become toxic with heavy metals, which are ingested by the fish we eat. Generally larger fish, like tuna, will be higher in toxins than smaller fish, although where the fish are harvested will also dictate levels of toxicity.

Legumes are an excellent food and also a source of protein, but they do not, by themselves, provide the complete balance of amino acids required for health. Historically this problem had been solved by combining them with grains, but in the current state of carbohydrate intolerance that many people are experiencing, this may result in more carbohydrates than are optimal. When grains are used, quinoa, an ancient, and as yet unadulterated, grain makes an excellent selection. Quinoa, which is actually a seed, tends to be higher in protein than other grains and has not been subjected to the genetic modification that has altered so many other grains.

Sprouting foods increases protein content, and in the case of legumes, may make them more digestible.

When an animal is unable to metabolize and excrete toxins efficiently, many of these toxins will be stored in fat cells, suggesting that less fatty cuts of meat may be preferable. That having been said, some animal fat in the diet can be beneficial. Butter, for example, supplies a substance known as butyric acid, which has been shown to be protective against colon cancer.[51]

Another saturated fat that has been shown to have significant health benefits is coconut oil.[52,53] Coconut oil is probably the safest fat to use in cooking as it does not easily oxidize. Poly-unsaturated vegetable oils, such as safflower oil, sunflower oil, and others should not be used for cooking, as they oxidize quickly with heat, causing rancidity that can increase inflammation and toxemia. Olive oil, a monounsaturated fat, is also safer and can be used to cook at low to moderate temperatures. Olive oil has been used for generations by Mediterranean people, and has many health benefits.

Finally, most of the diet should consist of a wide variety of fresh fruits and vegetables.

Enhancing Digestion

The best food does little good if it cannot be properly digested and assimilated. Optimizing digestive function is as critical as the food we eat. Stress, genetically modified foods, intestinal parasites, some diseases, and pharmaceutical drugs such as anti-biotics, and proton pump inhibitors are some of the things that can interfere with optimal digestive function. A full discussion of digestive health is beyond the scope of a book that seeks to give an overview of treatment guidelines for a variety of conditions, but some discussion is essential.

When digestive function is suspected to be suboptimal, a number of symptoms can occur to suggest that we focus our attention to digestive function. Complaints of easy satiety, a sense of fullness in the stomach after eating, epigastric burning, belching, flatulence, bloating, abdominal cramps, loose, or irregular bowel movements, or constipation are some of the symptoms that suggest digestive stress. Sometimes patients will present with minimal gastro-intestinal (GI) symptoms, but may have chronically low iron or ferritin (a test that measures iron storage) levels, frequent infections, dark circles under the eyes, or osteoporosis due to malabsorption.

Generally some simple measures will correct the problem, leaving expensive testing for those patients who do not respond or for symptoms that suggest a possibly serious condition. Patients who are experiencing weight loss, blood in stools, black stools, or severe symptoms should seek medical care. Chronic diarrhea, loose stools, or bloating that is unresponsive to simple measures may indicate possible infestation of parasites in the intestine or other potentially serious condition.

A supplement of pancreatic enzymes 1 -2 capsules with each meal often helps enhance digestion and relieve symptoms. I usually reach for the bitter digestive herbs before using enzymes, as these herbs work to stimulate the flow of digestive juices and get things working normally again. However, enzymes will often end up giving the same result in the long run, as more efficient digestion provided by enzyme supplementation results in better nutrition to the digestive tract as well as other body systems. This increased nutrition in the digestive tract enhances healing such that enzyme supplementation is not required in the long run, unless the patient is elderly or has a more complicated picture.

When hydrochloric acid (stomach acid) deficiency is suspected, there may be epigastric fullness and difficulty in digesting proteins. The latter also suggests possible pancreatic enzyme deficiency as well.

Gentian root (Gentiana lutea) is specific for increasing the secretion of stomach acid as well as pancreatic enzyme output, and is especially indicated when a feeling of fullness occurs after eating, or there is a sense that the food just sits in the stomach for a long while. The root is a bitter digestive stimulant and is traditionally dispensed with ginger, which adds carminative, warming, and anti-inflammatory actions to the cooling and stimulating actions of the gentian. A dose 5 to 15 drops of gentian tincture taken 10 - 15 minutes before a meal often serves to alleviate symptoms of epigastric fullness fairly quickly.

As mentioned above, bitter herbs like gentian combine well with carminative herbs such as peppermint, ginger, fennel seed, or aniseed. A tincture of equal parts gentian and ginger, for example, might be dosed at 15 to 30 drops before meals.

Angelica archangelica, a Native American angelica, is another digestive bitter, but unlike gentian, Angelica is warming and contains carminative essential oils to prevent gas formation and balance the stimulating actions of the bitters. This is not the same plant as Angelica sinensis, also known as Chinese angelica or dong quai. Because Angelica archangelica already has carminative action, it is not necessary to add another carminative herb to balance the bitters.

Because digestive bitters stimulate the release of digestive juices from the stomach, pancreas and gall bladder, they prepare the digestive tract for the work of digestion and therefore do best if taken 10 - 15 minutes before meals. However the herbs work better when taken in the middle of meal than not at all!

One or two teaspoons of raw unpasteurized apple cider vinegar before meals can sometimes offer the simplest solution for enhancing digestion, especially when abdominal fullness follows a meal. The vinegar can be mixed in a small amount of water, ideally no more than an ounce. This will often work for mild HCL deficiency.

A trial of hydrochloric acid (HCL) can be initiated, if low HCL is suspected. The patient takes one capsule with each meal on the first day, increasing to two caps the second day, and so on, until a mild burning is experienced in the stomach. The number of capsules is then dropped back down to the pre-burning dose and continued as long as necessary. Doses should not exceed 5 capsules with each meal, even when symptoms of burning are not induced.

In most instances, herbs, pancreatic enzymes, or supplementation with HCL will eventually no longer be necessary as the digestive tract heals simply because nutrients are being absorbed and assimilated more efficiently. Some people will find a few months are all they need, while others will benefit from longer supplementation. Older patients may need lifelong supplementation of HCL as the cells that secrete HCL can atrophy as we grow older.

Paradoxical as it may seem, epigastric burning can occur as a result of low HCL. An overly alkaline environment is just as likely to cause burning as an over abundance of acid. In these cases, one or two teaspoons of apple cider vinegar before meals may be the gentlest place to start. If this is well tolerated or brings relief, Gentian or HCL may be the next step.

Vitamin B12 may also be deficient if HCL is low, as the parietal cells in the stomach which secrete HCL also secrete a substance called intrinsic factor which is essential for the absorption of vitamin B12. If HCL deficiency is due to atrophy of parietal cells, vitamin B12 may need to be given intra-muscularly as oral doses may not be absorbed.

A simple CBC (complete blood count) can be run to assess MCV levels, which may be high in B12 deficiency. While the MCV can be normal in some patients with vitamin B12 deficiency, generally, an MCV over 90 - 95 is suggestive in the symptomatic patient while a level over 100 is more definitely diagnostic. Serum levels of Vitamin B12 are not considered particularly useful by most holistic practitioners as symptoms of B12 deficiency are often seen with normal serum levels of B12.

A more recent test to consider for evaluation of vitamin B12 status is methylmalonic acid which is highly sensitive for B12 deficiency. Because vitamin B12 is essential for the breakdown of methylmalonic acid to succinyl-CoA, elevated levels of methylmalonic acid are strongly suggestive of a vitamin B12 deficiency especially when homocysteine levels are also elevated.[54]

If B12 deficiency is chronic and associated with atrophy of parietal cells in the stomach, as can occur with aging, a diagnosis may be made of pernicious anemia, a macrocytic anemia (anemia with enlarged red blood cells).

Despite the fact that this water soluble vitamin does store in the liver, the once per month regimen sometimes prescribed by allopathic practitioners has not always appeared to be adequate in my clinical experience. While this lower dosage strategy may be enough to correct anemia, it does not appear to be adequate to assure optimal health. The elders who are the most vulnerable group of patients to develop pernicious anemia report better mental functioning with more frequent doses of intra-muscular B12.

To help increase liver stores of vitamin B 12, I usually start with an injection of 1000 micrograms 2 - 3 times per week for a week or two, then go to once per week following patient symptoms as well as lab indices. Mental functioning will be the best guide for many of these patients. Patients who are struggling with chronic fatigue, nerve pain, or paresthesias (odd sensations due to malfunction or impingement of nerves) may also benefit from additional B 12. Vitamin B 12 is vital for phase II methylation pathways of detoxification, in which case we may be utilizing more of the vitamin than we did before our environment became so toxic.

For more information on dosing strategies for injectable vitamin B12, please refer to the discussion in the chapter on musculoskeletal conditions.

Oral Thrush

Thrush is a condition common to childhood. A white creamy plaque covering parts of the oral cavity, particularly the tongue or buccal mucosa (inner cheeks) is caused by an overgrowth of the fungus, Candida albicans. Lesions tend to bleed when disturbed and are usually easy to scrape off. The condition can be painful, causing the child to be reluctant to nurse or take food.

Although less common in adults, thrush can sometimes be seen in patients who are run down, have recently been through a course of anti-biotics, or are using steroid inhalers. It can also occur as a result of an immunodeficiency state such as HIV, or cancer.

Simple thrush is nearly always responsive to treatment with homeopathic Pulsatilla. A 30C potency given four times per day is usually effective. Anti-fungal herbs, such as Echinacea, Chilopsis, Spilanthes, or Usnea can also be given to help build up the immune system and prevent further episodes. A tea of the herbs used should be swished in the mouth before swallowing to provide a local effect.

Dental abscess

Dental abscesses should be evaluated by a dentist but unless the tooth is rotten, the acute infection can usually be cleared up easily with a well selected homeopathic remedy.

Mercurius is a common remedy for the truly acute infection. When this remedy is indicated, there will be excessive salivation and halitosis (bad breath).

Silica will suit the patient whose abscess is more low grade and chronic.

While other remedies, including the appropriate constitutional remedy, may be indicated, Mercurius and Silica have been most common in my practice.

If the teeth are rotten, and the patient presents with fever, chills and malaise, homeopathic Pyrogen should be considered. Extraction of the rotten tooth will be necessary in these cases to completely eradicate infection.

Echinacea root is my top herb for abscesses of any sort, as it acts as a lymphatic and blood cleanser as well an immune-modulator. In more serious cases, Baptisia tinctoria should be added in as it is specific for infection with toxemia and enhances the actions of Echinacea.

For patients with a chronic tendency to abscesses anywhere in the body, blood cleansers such as Trifolium, Arctium, Urtica, Scrophularia, and Ceanothus should be considered in addition to the Echinacea. Flavonoid rich foods, such as dark colored berries and beets will also be helpful in clearing toxins and providing nutrients to decrease inflammation and encourage healing. Attention to the state of the liver will also be important in these cases.

Echinacea can be dosed freely, with tincture doses going up to 60 drops every two hours. Baptisia, however, has potential toxicity and should be dosed more conservatively. An average adult dose of a 1:1 fresh herb tincture of Baptisia may be dosed at 10 drops 4 times per day.

Gastro-esophageal Reflux (GERD) and Epigastric Burning

Etiologies and differential diagnoses for GERD and gastric or esophageal burning should be considered. Persistent symptoms should be worked up. It is also important to remember that an acute myocardial infarction (heart attack) can mask as heartburn, usually with a sense of pressure in the chest. Persistent or worsening symptoms could indicate cancer or ulceration. Black or tarry stools are strongly suggestive of bleeding in the upper intestinal tract and the patient should be evaluated thoroughly if these symptoms are present. The following are a few simple things that have worked when symptoms are straightforward and uncomplicated by more serious conditions. These suggestions are often efficacious in providing a nourishing baseline for the treatment of more serious conditions as well.

Nourishing and rebuilding protective mucous membrane surfaces is vital for protecting underlying tissues from inflammation. A gruel of powdered Althea officinalis (marshmallow root) can be taken by the tablespoon as often as every 5 - 10 minutes when needed during acute episodes of burning, dropping to 4 to 8 times per day for ongoing healing and repair of mucosal tissues.

Another herb, more commonly prescribed as a mucous membrane demulcent and readily available on the market in health food stores is slippery elm bark. Although harvesting the roots of Althea necessitates killing the whole plant, Althea is an easily cultivated and attractive weed that grows quickly and abundantly, while slippery elm comes from the bark of a tree, which takes many years to grow. Please use Althea. The use of slippery elm bark, while effective, is really not as ecologically responsible.

Classic Recipe for Althea Gruel

1) Slowly stir 1/4 cup of cold juice or water into 1.5 to 2 teaspoons of powdered Althea root to make a paste.
2) Add 1.5 to 2 cups of boiling water or juice, stirring for two minutes.
3) Cinnamon, raisins, honey, or other seasonings may be added for flavor.
4) Alternatively, doses of the gruel can be added to foods such as oatmeal.

Gruel should be taken several times per day to heal mucous membranes of digestive, respiratory, or urinary tracts. When epigastric burning or intestinal inflammation flares, 1 tablespoon or more of gruel can be taken every few minutes as needed. Because the herb is completely nontoxic, simply sipping the herb continuously throughout the day is safe and may be more efficacious than taking a larger dose less often. Sharol Tilgner (Medicines from the Heart of the Earth) recommends doses of up to 6 cups per day. Althea has also proven helpful in the treatment of severe dry eyes associated with underlying immune dysfunction.

Glycerrhiza glabra, licorice root, (see chapter on adaptogens) is an excellent choice for the treatment of inflammatory conditions of the digestive tract. Licorice acts to modulate inflammation and enhance immune function through adreno-cortical mechanisms as well as provide demulcent, mucilaginous nourishment to heal and rebuild mucous membranes. Adaptogenic qualities may help tonify stress responses that are contributing to symptoms.

The inner gel of the aloe vera plant provides a highly mucilaginous that has often proven useful in alleviating symptoms of burning and irritation in the GI tract. The juice or gel may be dosed at 1 - 2 tablespoons 1 - 3 times per day.

An old naturopathic/herbal compound, known as Robert's Formula, combines several herbs to facilitate healing in the GI tract. While there seem to be several versions of Robert's Formula these days, the basic formula includes a combination of demulcent herbs, (Ulmus, Althea, okra), blood cleansing anti-microbials, (Echinacea, Baptisia, Hydrastis), astringents, (Geranium) and lymphatics (Phytolacca).

Symphytum officinalis, comfrey root and leaf, is a highly demulcent herb with powerful constituents to promote healing. When used topically to promote wound healing, care must be taken to be sure there is no infection, as comfrey will heal the tissue so quickly it can potentially heal an infection in.

Internal use of comfrey was once popular and highly efficacious for GI conditions with inflammation and disruption of mucous membranes. Unfortunately, this herb tends to be rich in pyrrolizidine alkaloids,[55] which break down to an intermediary in the liver that has been shown to cause severe, irreversible veno-occlusive liver disease in some individuals.

Patients who have compromise in phase II pathways of detoxification may be at higher risk of problems with these particular alkaloids, as it is thought that the initial breakdown product of pyrrolizidine alkaloids, the intermediary created from the first phase of detoxification, is actually what is causing the problem, not the alkaloids themselves.

These intermediaries are meant to be immediately picked up and inactivated by phase II pathways, but unfortunately today phase II pathways are often overloaded and unable to hold up to the demand that our modern environment inflicts on us. As seems to be the case with the pyrrolizidine alkaloids, some of the intermediaries coming out of the first phase of detoxification are more toxic than the original substance.

Our ancestors, whose detoxification pathways were not overwhelmed by the enormous levels of toxins that are ubiquitous in the world today, were more easily able to break down pyrrolizidine alkaloids, thus avoiding any potential dangers. The problem appears to be not in the plant, but in our toxic environment and consequent congested pathways of detoxification. For this reason, internal use of comfrey, even in the short term, is no longer advised.

Cabbage juice has been shown to be useful in repairing the integrity of the GI tract. In one clinical trial in which a group of prisoners were given a quart of cabbage juice each day, healing of peptic ulcers was seen on imaging within 22 days.[56] Use of the juice provides cancer preventing anthocyanidins as well as other health benefits. In studies, cabbage juice has been dosed at 1 cup 4 times per day. Smaller doses may also provide benefit however, especially when used in conjunction with other therapies.

Avoidance of substances that aggravate symptoms, such as coffee, tobacco, gluten, dairy and other individual sensitivities is vital, as continued ingestion of offending substances can create an obstacle to healing. Peppermint should be avoided in patients with gastroesophageal reflux as it tends to aggravate the problem by relaxing the sphincter at the juncture of the esophagus and the stomach.

Although these are chronic cases in which any number of homeopathic remedies may be indicated, Pulsatilla is very commonly helpful. Other remedies I have seen be of help include Calcarea carbonica (the over-responsible worrier), Arsenicum album (fearful and anxious), and Argentum nitricum (stomach symptoms from overexcitement).

Liver

The liver is central to maintaining and establishing optimal health, as it is the main organ of detoxification. This organ also plays an important role in many other metabolic processes, including blood sugar regulation, digestion and metabolism of fats, proteins and carbohydrates, and hormone regulation.

In the past, therapeutic fasting was often utilized as a tool to facilitate detoxification. Fasting on diluted juices, vegetable broths, and herbal teas, rather than just water, can provide nutrients to neutralize acidic toxins, allowing for easier excretion of toxins and more efficient detoxification. Fasting is not as well tolerated today, except in those folks who are still fortunate enough to enjoy robust vitality. Most patients seeking help with detoxification are experiencing too much endocrine stress from environmental toxins for fasting to be therapeutic. Fasting can be detrimental in these cases, as the body struggles to maintain adequate blood sugar levels without regular ingestion of food.

Because our environment is flooded with an unprecedented amount of toxins, the topic of detoxification has become much more complex. Heavy metals, such as lead and mercury, for example, require more specific protocols for elimination. Basic detoxification protocols still hold true however, and simple protocols that involve cleansing diets, fiber, enemas, saunas, massage, dry skin brushing, and ingestion of nutritional or herbal products that offer support and key constituents necessary for optimal detoxification are still highly efficacious.[57]

Our livers benefit greatly from changing the way we eat. Simply stopping junk food, greasy food, sweets, sodas, and processed foods lightens the load on the liver so that detoxification can take place normally again. Adding in good quality proteins, an abundance of dark green leafy vegetables, Brassica family vegetables, colorful vegetables, and plenty of fresh fruit can be huge in helping the liver to detox. In fact there really is little point in doing a "liver cleanse" unless you plan to follow it up with a diet and lifestyle changes aimed to keep you healthy.

Adequate amounts of good quality water are also essential for toxins to be washed out of tissues and carried through the kidneys, sweat, lungs, and colon for elimination.

Herbs that nourish and protect the liver or stimulate liver function can be very helpful for detoxification, and I have often seen liver enzymes come back to normal when a formula of one or more of these herbs has been given in conjunction with dietary changes. Liver enzyme levels are tested on a metabolic panel, which is done on routine blood draws. Liver enzymes are elevated in the presence of ongoing injury to liver cells.

Elevations in cholesterol (over 200 to 220) can be an indicator of liver congestion, as cholesterol is largely synthesized in the liver.[58] The primary use of cholesterol in the liver is for the production of cholic acid which is conjugated to produce bile salts. These bile salts are then secreted into the duodenum for digestion of fats, making the gall bladder and colon primary routes for the excretion of cholesterol from the body.[59]

Knowledge of this basic biochemistry has led me to treat the liver whenever cholesterol is elevated and in the early days of my practice, the use of bitter liver herbs in combination with dietary changes was all that was necessary to lower abnormally high levels of cholesterol. Although I still treat the liver as the primary organ in hyperlipidemia, patients do not respond as quickly as they once did, probably again due to increased environmental toxicity.

Statin drugs, which are commonly prescribed to lower cholesterol, have been associated with increases in liver enzymes in some patients. Because elevated liver enzymes are a sign of hepatocellular injury, these drugs may well be stressing the very organ that needs to be treated. In any case, statins do not address underlying causes.

Cholesterol is essential in the production of various hormones, including testosterone, estrogen, progesterone and adrenocortical hormones, making adequate levels of cholesterol vital for optimal endocrine function.[60]

Elevations in cholesterol are also seen in hypo-thyroidism. Treatment of low thyroid function will normalize cholesterol levels in the absence of other mitigating factors in these cases.

Extreme elevations in cholesterol (400+) may be indicative of acute kidney disease. These patients should be worked up for the presence of renal disease as soon as possible, so treatment to prevent progression to renal failure can be instituted promptly. There are a number of herbs that have been shown to be renal-protective and restorative to glomerular function, with Salvia miltiorrhiza, Panax ginseng, Ginkgo biloba, Silybum marianum, and Zea mays being a few. As important organs of filtration and elimination, the kidneys are also prone to be stressed by increased environmental toxicity.

It is generally wise to avoid strong liver herbs in patients who present with low vitality, blocked emunctories, or significant environmental sensitivities. Many patients who present with environmental sensitivities appear to have compromise in Phase II enzyme systems, either from nutritional deficiencies or toxic overload. In these cases, it is most prudent to begin with lifestyle and dietary alterations, accompanied by liver rebuilding and nourishing herbs, such as Silybum marianum (milk thistle seed), Glycerrhiza glabra (licorice root), Curcuma longa (turmeric), Hypericum perfoliatum (St. John's Wort), Salvia miltitorrhiza (Chinese sage root), Schisandra chinesis, Ceanothus spp. and many others.

Foods that are particularly useful to the liver include beets and beet greens, dark green leafy vegetables, and artichokes. Beets contain catechins, a type of flavonoid shown to be particularly protective to the liver. Beets also help optimize bile flow from the gall bladder into the small intestine, promoting drainage of the liver and further enhancing elimination of toxins. Onions, garlic, legumes, eggs, and members of the Brassicaceae or cabbage family are high in sulfur and help support phase II detoxification. Adequate good quality protein is essential for optimal live function.

Silybum marianum, milk thistle seed, is protective and restorative to both liver and kidney. Silybum is rich in antioxidant, anti-inflammatory flavonoids and is thought to be a powerful precursor to the production of glutathione, an important substance created by the body to protect cells from oxidative damage initiated by toxic reactions.

Salvia miltiorrhiza is protective to the kidneys, liver, and heart. In my clinical practice, it has proven to be an excellent herb for renal stress or early renal failure to return glomerular function to normal, or in later stages, to delay the need for dialysis.

Once a patient's channels of elimination are working well and their vitality has improved, I will often prescribe a formula of herbs that stimulate liver function more actively and promote drainage from the liver, gall bladder, and colon. If the patient's vitality or ability to handle toxins has been compromised in the recent past, as is often seen with environmentally sensitive patients, I may start with a tea of dandelion. One half to 1 teaspoon of chopped root is decocted for 10 minutes then poured over 1/2 to 1 teaspoon of leaf. This can be taken three times per day, or in the less vital or more sensitive patient, the preparation can be divided into three doses, preferably ingesting 1/3 of the tea before each meal to enhance digestion.

The bright yellow flowers of the ever optimistic dandelion (Taraxacum officinalis) burst up each spring like smiley bundles of sunshine, reminding us that spring has traditionally been a time for cleansing and renewal. The whole plant should be used, with the root being more specific for the liver and gall bladder and the leaf acting as a diuretic to aid elimination through the kidney. The herb is also nutritious to the liver.

For the more vital patient, a formula of herbs such as Chelidonium, Mahonia spp., Chionanthus, and Bupleurum, may be combined in formula with Cynara, Taraxacum, Silybum, and Curcumin with good effects. An average dose of such a formula might be 15 - 30 drops 3 times per day. Start low and work up as tolerated.

Because these stimulating herbs release toxins back into the bloodstream to be eliminated through the kidneys, lungs, and skin as well as through the colon, the formula should be discontinued if acute symptoms occur, such as a cold or flu, urinary tract infection, headache, or significant skin rash. These acute conditions suggest that the body is temporarily discharging more toxins than the channels of elimination can handle without becoming symptomatic. Such pathologic symptom pictures are not necessarily a negative thing, but often represent a healing crisis, wherein the body has elected to discharge an increased amount of toxins. In these cases, the liver stimulating herbs should be stopped while the acute process is supported through appropriate herbs, homeopathics, or hydrotherapy. Saunas, colonics or enemas, daily dry skin brushing with a loofah sponge, and deep breathing in fresh county air will help enhance elimination while liver stimulating herbs are being taken.

Gall Bladder

Classic symptoms of acute gall bladder inflammation (cholecystitis) include a sharp or aching pain in the RUQ (right upper quadrant) of the abdomen, just lateral to the midline where the gall bladder is tucked under the liver. Pain can radiate to the back where it classically causes an ache under the right clavicle (shoulder blade).

In actual practice, cholecystitis can manifest as generalized abdominal pain, or may mimic symptoms of GERD, angina, or myocardial infarction (heart attack) with burning or pressure under the sternum. Often there will be loss of appetite, nausea, and sometimes constipation. Pain can be anywhere in the abdomen and will sometimes present as generalized abdominal pain or with localization to other parts of the abdomen, making differential diagnosis important to avoid missing an acute appendicitis or other serious abdominal conditions.

When gall bladder disease is suspected, the physician examines the abdomen by pressing three fingers up under the rib cage just to the right of the midline as the patient inhales deeply. Gall bladder involvement can be strongly suspected if an increase in pain occurs on deep inspiration, which causes the gall bladder to be pushed against the pressure of the physician's hand.

Blood work may or may not show elevations in bilirubin in chronic cholecystitis. Significant elevations in liver enzymes should suggest underlying liver pathology or acute cholangitis. If the patient is passing a gall stone through the common bile duct, liver enzymes may be elevated due to blockage of the common bile duct causing a backflow of bile into the liver. These latter patients will usually be in significant pain.

Abdominal ultrasounds (US) are commonly ordered for evaluation of the gall bladder. US may show thickening of the wall of the gall bladder and presence of stones but may or may not show positive findings in the presence of cholecystitis.

Gall bladder disease appears to be on the increase. While it was once seen as a disease of middle aged women, generally forty years of age and over, it is now occurring in younger people as well. This increased incidence is probably related to the increased stress on the liver which is responsible for producing all the bile that goes into the gall bladder.

Bitter herbs used for gall bladder disease can act as cholagogues, choloretics or both. Cholagogues stimulate the flow of bile into the duodenum, while choleretics stimulate the liver to produce bile. These bitter herbs all affect liver and digestive function in varying degrees.

Most bitters also stimulate intestinal peristalsis, ensuring adequate elimination through the colon while stimulating the liver to process toxins more efficiently. Unlike too many modern physicians, these simple plants seem to know that gall bladders cannot be healed without also attending to the health of the liver.

Attention to the diet is critical for anyone suffering with gall bladder symptoms. Rich, fried, and fatty foods must be eliminated, and replaced with a moderate amount of healthy fats such as olive oil, avocados, coconut oil, fatty wild caught fish, and fish oils. Some patients in more acute disease may have difficulty tolerating even small amounts of healthy fats. The key here is to follow the body's wisdom and keep fat and oil intake to the minimum required to avoid symptoms, adding good fats in as healing progresses and the patient is again able to tolerate them in the diet.

Other foods that should be kept minimal or eliminated in the acute phase include poultry and eggs, as these foods can be irritating to the gall bladder. Some patients will find that garlic and possibly onions are also not well tolerated when the gall bladder is acutely inflamed. The long term goal, of course, is to have these healthy foods reintroduced into the diet but kept in moderation. Greasy fried foods are not healthy for any of us, and rich fatty foods should also be kept out of the diet if the patient wants to stay healthy and avoid further flare ups of gall bladder inflammation.

Homeopathy, herbs and Chinese Medicine are all very powerful modalities for healing gall bladder inflammation and can often subvert the need for surgery. In addition, castor oil packs applied to the entire abdomen will help relieve pain, reduce inflammation, and increase circulation to the digestive tract as well as the liver and gall bladder.

When patients present with symptoms suggestive of acute or subacute cholecystitis, a simple prescription of homeopathic Chelidonium will often serve to heal the acute crisis. If the patient with abdominal pain is positive for pain in the right upper quadrant, and reports that symptoms are worse with fatty foods, Chelidonium 30C given four times daily will often bring significant relief.

Once the patient is out of the acute phase, or if symptoms are not severe at onset, herbs to stimulate bile flow (cholagogues) may be initiated. Some of these herbs are also choloretics and will stimulate the liver to produce bile. The bitter herbs used to treat cholecystitis (inflammation of the gall bladder) or cholestasis (sluggish gall bladder function) also increase digestive function and promote peristalsis to prevent constipation.

Chelidonium majus (Greater Celandine), the herb from which the homeopathic remedy is derived, is perhaps one of our strongest cholagogues. Other fairly strong cholagogues include, but are not limited to, Chionanthus virginicus (fringe tree), Taraxacum officinialis (dandelion root), and Mahonia spp. (Oregon grape root).

Some alteratives such as Iris versicolor (blue flag), and Baptisia tinctoria (wild indigo) can also act as cholagogues.

Finally, simple herbs such as the culinary Rosemarinus officianalis (rosemary) and the popular Mentha piperita (peppermint leaves) can also be of service in stimulating bile flow without being as potentially overstimulating as Chelidonium or Chionanthus might be for some patients.

Persistent or severe symptoms of abdominal pain or discomfort should not be treated lightly. Gall stones that are being passed through the common bile duct (the channel that carries bile from the gall bladder to the duodenum) into the duodenum can get lodged and block the pancreatic duct causing a severe condition known as pancreatitis. This condition can only be assessed by a qualified medical practitioner, who may elect to do imaging and/or draw blood to check levels of liver enzymes, bilirubin, lipase, and amylase. Liver enzymes allow the practitioner to assess and evaluate the degree of stress the liver may be undergoing as a result of blocked bile flow, while serum amylase and lipase aid in assessing pancreatic stress. An elevation in either serum amylase or lipase should be a red flag for the naturopathic practitioner to refer for surgery. Despite a recent trend towards running only a lipase, I have seen at least one case where an acute pancreatitis was missed by the gastroenterologist when a serum amylase was not run and lipase was normal. When blood was drawn in our clinic, the amylase it was significantly elevated, confirming our suspicion of acute pancreatitis.

Although uncommon, acute cholangitis, an infectious or toxic condition of the common bile duct, is a very serious condition and must be treated promptly by a qualified medical health care provider. In these cases, gall bladder pain is accompanied by fever and chills and the patient will be very ill. There may be jaundice and possibly mental confusion. Liver enzymes and white blood cell count will be elevated. Cholangitis usually involves a bacterial infection and differs from cholecystitis which is an inflammatory condition and not an infection. Cholangitis can quickly progress to septic shock if left untreated.

The common practice of performing a supposed "gall stone cleanse" is reputed to stimulate the gall bladder to pass gall stones into the stool. This method uses varying but fairly large amounts of olive oil and lemon juice, taken either in one large dose in the morning or at slightly more moderate doses every 15 minutes or so. This practice is controversial and it is highly doubtful that it actually stimulates the release of gall stones into the intestinal tract. Evaluation of material that is passed in the stool has not been proven to be gall stones. In addition, if this treatment were working in the way it claims, with the passing of the large amount of stones the treatment claims to provoke, it would very likely lead to a gall bladder colic, with some of the stones potentially getting trapped in the common bile duct causing significant spasm and pain. Some of us, myself included, have seen patients put themselves into acute cholangitis using this treatment. Despite claims, the intense olive oil lemon juice "cleanse" is just not a good idea.

Colon

Because the large intestine is a primary emunctory for the elimination of toxins, an unhealthy colon can be a contributory factor in any illness. Constipation allows stool to sit in the colon overlong facilitating the reabsorption of toxins that should be leaving the body. Diarrhea or loose stools may reflect parasitic infestation, malabsorption, dysbiosis, or inflammatory bowel disease. Excess intestinal gas may be due to poor digestion. Abdominal bloating may be due to a buildup of gas in the intestines or stagnation in the lymphatic mesentery that surrounds the intestine. Dysbiosis or lymphatic stagnation can also contribute to immune stress.

Simple constipation should first be treated with dietary fiber, adequate water intake, and regular exercise. Beets have laxative properties and can be especially helpful if constipation is due to gall bladder stasis. If simple measures are not adequate, supplemental magnesium can be taken in doses of 200 - 300 milligrams every 2 hours until results are obtained. Laxative herbs containing anthroquinone glycosides, such as Senna leaves and Cascara stimulate peristalsis, but can also cause cramping and griping in the intestine if the dose is too high. They are usually reserved as a last resort, as simple lifestyle modifications usually do the trick. When they are used I have usually found the tea to be most efficacious.

Good quality probiotics cannot be underestimated in restoring healthy function to the colon.[61] While many people are aware of the importance of Lactobacillus spp., another probiotic, Saccharomyces boulardii, is also important, due to its ability to colonize the colon, prevent Candida overgrowth, and enhance the growth and colonization of favorable intestinal bacteria. Because Saccharomyces is a yeast, it will not be affected by anti-biotics, which only go after bacteria. For this reason, Saccharomyces should always be given with a prescription of anti-biotics, to prevent dysbiosis and overgrowth of Candida.

Saccharomyces is specific for treating Clostridium difficile, a potentially serious infection in the intestines that may occur after the use of certain anti-biotics.

Saccharomyces should be given during the entire course of anti-biotic treatment and for 2 - 4 weeks afterwards, whereas Lactobacillus spp. may need to be continued for several months, depending on the situation.

Lactobacillus reuterii and L. rhamnosus may be of specific aid in patients with bacterial vaginosis.[62]

Finally the condition commonly known as irritable bowel syndrome (IBS), responds well to improvements in diet and elimination of offending foods, particularly gluten and possibly dairy as well. For patients who suffer from excessive flatulence and bloating, a carminative formula of 1/2 peppermint, 1/4 aniseed, and 1/4 fennel seed can be dispensed in tincture with doses of 15 drops 3 times per day often being optimal.

Alternatively a tea of equal parts of chamomile, licorice, fennel seed, and peppermint can be dosed at 1 tablespoon per cup, 2 - 4 cups per day.

The peppermint in both formulas adds antispasmodic, anti-inflammatory and bitters to the carminative actions. Chamomile is carminative, anti-spasmodic and anti-inflammatory in the intestinal tract, and helps sooth irritated nerves as well. Licorice adds demulcent, anti-inflammatory and adrenal adaptogenic properties.

The addition of constitutional homeopathic prescribing can bring wonderful relief to these patients.

Chapter 8
Chronic Fatigue Syndrome

CHRONIC FATIGUE CAN BE CAUSED by a variety of problems, including but not limited to, low thyroid function, chronic viral infection, lyme disease, anemia, autoimmune disease, cardiovascular disease, dysglycemia, intestinal parasites, heavy metal toxicity or cancer. It is therefore important to rule out etiologies that may be causing fatigue or aggravating any underlying viral pathology. Although viral titers may be helpful in confirming suspicions of infection, these tests are not always conclusive and chronic viral diseases, such as cytomegalo virus (CMV), chronic herpes virus (HSV), and Epstein Barr virus (EBV) are often a diagnosis of exclusion. In any case these viruses thrive best in toxic soil, making constitutional work and treatment of susceptibility and toxicity paramount for these patients.

Although any comment on mental emotional patterns can only be taken as a generality, it does seem that chronic fatigue symptoms flare when personal power is challenged or the patient lacks the ability to stand in their power.

There are many cultural taboos and much confusion about personal power with women often taking too much responsibility for the feelings of others or getting trapped in the cultural pressure to "be nice" even when circumstances might dictate that being nice is likely to get them hammered.

Men on the other hand may reject their fire in order to avoid being associated with patriarchal abuse. One young man shared with me many years ago that whenever he spoke from his power or expressed any fieriness in his voice, he felt haunted by the looks of fear in the eyes of the women around him.

Claiming personal power is always something of an edge. Certainly we do not want our patients to become overbearing and abusive. Classes in something like nonviolent communication (NVC), originally formulated by Dr. Marshal Rosenberg, can be very helpful in facilitating effective communication that does not batter or criticize another person.

The consistent incidence of liver congestion in patients with chronic fatigue syndrome confirms an association between our increasingly toxic environment and the rising incidence of fibromyalgia and chronic viral disease. Data going as far back as the 1980s shows that exposure to environmental toxins decreases immune response, rendering us more susceptible to viral infections.[63] Here is an instance where naturopathic philosophy is well illustrated. It is not the virus itself that causes disease but rather the toxicity of the terrain (the patient's body) that determines susceptibility to microbial invasion and subsequent illness.

Liver enzymes may be mildly elevated in these patients and liver tenderness on palpation is a common finding. In addition, patients with chronic viral diseases commonly report some degree of hypersensitivity to environmental toxins, such as perfumes, new carpets, and even newsprint. Although severe chemical hypersensitivity is not limited to patients with chronic viral syndromes, these patients are more prone to develop crippling chemical intolerances. Treatment with pharmaceutical medications simply does not make sense for a patient population already compromised in their ability to break down chemical toxins. Treatment of underlying toxicity, on the other hand, renders the body's terrain less friendly to viral invasion. The patient's environment should be as free of chemical toxins as possible. Testing for and then treating any heavy metal toxicity should also be considered.

Adrenal, liver, and immune support are essential in treating these patients. In addition, constitutional homeopathy or acupuncture will do much to stimulate the patient's vitality.

When selecting adaptogenic herbs, plants that are also anti-viral, such as licorice or holy basil, may be preferred. Cat's claw, with its high flavonoid content, will work doubly well at reducing inflammation, particularly when fibromyalgia is a part of the patient picture. Cat's claw and licorice are also hepatoprotective.

Highly sensitive patients will generally not do well on liver stimulating herbs such as Chelidonium (greater celandine) or Chionanthus (fringe tree) and many sensitive patients will even experience reactions with Taraxacum (dandelion) or Chinese Bupleurum.

It is generally a good idea to start with liver nourishing, hepatoprotective herbs such as turmeric and milk thistle, both of which are generally well tolerated. Licorice and Schisandra may also be of help as hepatoprotective herbs as well as adaptogens.

I often dose turmeric as a powder and suggest patients take 1/2 teaspoon twice daily. Environmentally sensitive patients may find that an extra 1/2 teaspoon dose as needed decreases symptoms after inadvertent exposure to toxins.

Despite recent claims that turmeric is not easily absorbed in the digestive tract, whole turmeric actually contains bitter principles that aid in digestion. I have had good results clinically using whole powdered herb.

Milk thistle seeds can be taken in fairly high doses and will be less expensive as a powder than in tincture or capsules. Because the seeds contain oils that easily oxidize and become rancid, it is best to buy whole seeds and grind them in a coffee grinder as needed. Any left over ground seed should be refrigerated and used within a few days. Usual dosage recommendations are 1 - 2 tablespoons of powdered herb per day. Milk thistle is highly active as a precursor to glutathione,[64] an important antioxidant made by the body to handle toxins and enhance immune function.

A diet high in a variety of vegetables and adequate protein is essential for optimal liver function. Onions, garlic, and brassica family vegetables such as cabbage, broccoli, kale, and cauliflower will provide sulfur compounds for phase two sulfonation pathways of detoxification. Beets and beet greens provide catechins and flavonoids that are hepato-protective, while the beet roots encourage drainage of the gall bladder, which allows toxins to drain from the liver as well. Dark green leafy vegetables are also ideal. Foods and herbs high in anthocyanin, such as blueberries, dark grapes, pomegranate seeds, rose hips, hawthorne, or cherries will help aid in tying up toxic reactions in the body and decrease inflammation.

Castor oil packs can be used over the abdomen for twenty minutes in the evening to decrease inflammation and mobilize stagnation in the liver and lymphatic mesentery surrounding the intestines. A piece of organic cotton or wool that has not been dyed or bleached should be moistened with the castor oil and warmed in the oven to a tolerable temperature. The size of the cloth should be large enough to cover the abdomen from the rib cage to the pubic bone. The pack is laid on the abdomen and covered with a hot water bottle to keep it warm. As the castor oil permanently stains any clothing it contacts, an old tee shirt and pair of sweat pants should be reserved just for the occasion.

Immune enhancing herbs such as licorice, osha, lomatium, astragalus, and echinacea should also be considered. Lymphatic support may be important, especially if infection with Epstein Barr Virus (EBV) is part of the picture. Since this particular virus affects the spleen as well as the liver, a tincture of Ceanothus, 15 drops three times per day, will help support liver, lymph, and spleen function.

In some cases, symptoms of fibromyalgia may be relieved by small doses of an herbal tincture of Arnica montana. This herb has potential for toxicity, so proper dosage is critical. Six drops three times per day has worked well for the occasional fibromyalgia patient, and while it does not work all the time, one patient's pain was completely cured by the herbal tincture of Arnica.

Arnica is contraindicated if there is gastrointestinal inflammation. Symptoms of toxicity include nervous unrest, agitation, and gastric irritation. Death from significant overdose can result due to cardiac arrest.

Some patients will experience temporary relief of fibromyalgia pains with a combination of kava, black cohosh, and Jamaican dogwood taken in small doses throughout the day.

The most reliable treatment I have found for fibromyalgia, however, has been homeopathic Rhus tox 30C taken 2 - 4 times per day, with the last dose always at bedtime. The remedy may be repeated if the patient wakes with pain during the night.

As symptoms improve, the Rhus tox should be taken less often perhaps 2 or 3 times instead of 4. It is important that the dose at bedtime be discontinued last as the pain of fibromyalgia is often aggravated by rest and worse in the morning on rising.

Many times the correctly selected constitutional remedy alone will relieve pains of fibromyalgia, in which case, other measures are unnecessary. But often the pain persists, in which case Rhus tox can be added in along with the constitutional remedy.

Because the pain of fibromyalgia often prevents even moderate exercise, interferes with sleep, and frequently drives the patient to the use of such medicaments as ibuprofen or low dose naltrexone, it is important to relieve the pain and the underlying stagnation in the tissues for optimal healing to occur.

Chapter 9

Conditions of the Respiratory Tract

MILK AND MILK PRODUCTS such as cheese and yogurt are generally aggravating to respiratory conditions. These foods should be discontinued from the diet whether the respiratory complaint is acute or chronic. Once the acute condition has resolved patients may be able to return milk products to the diet unless there is a tendency to frequent episodes.

SINUSITIS

Acute sinusitis responds well to a tincture of equal parts of horse radish (Amoracia rusticana) and yerba mansa (Anemopsis californica) administered together at a dose of 60 drops 5 - 10 times per day. The addition of the peppery horseradish stimulates mucous membranes of the sinuses and nasal passages, loosening up thick mucous, decreasing congestion and relieving pain as a result. For this reason a few drops of each dose should ideally be taken directly onto the tongue to facilitate the drainage effects of the horseradish. Horseradish also has some anti-microbial activity.

Homeopathic remedies that most often prove helpful for acute sinusitis are Mercurius vivus (Merc) and Kali bichromicum (Kali bich).

Symptoms calling for Kali bich include pain and pressure at the base of the nose. There is often the feeling that blocked mucous sits like a brick in the sinus cavity. Watery discharge may be absent, scanty, or profuse. Thicker discharge may occur as plugs of mucous or thick ropy yellowish green mucous. Discharge, if present, does not relieve the sensation of pressure and mucous buildup in the sinus cavities.

The Mercurius sinusitis often presents with more discharge, which is generally excoriating. There may be a sense of rawness and burning in sinus cavities. Nasal discharge will usually be more profuse and free flowing than patients who need Kali bich, although a thick discharge may also be seen. Both remedies can have watery or yellowish green discharge. An increase in salivation is almost always present when Mercurius is the remedy, and there may be a tendency to drool on the pillow at night. Sneezing is common.

Homeopathic Sticta, prepared from the lichen Lobaria pulmonaria, once known as Sticta pulmonaria, may be used in cases where Kali bich seems indicated but does not work. This remedy is less common, but is worth knowing for those rare times when it is indicated. There is a sense of dryness in the nasal passages, with fullness at the base of the nose. Despite a persistent desire to blow the nose, no discharge appears. In cases due to hay fever, the patient will be bothered by constant sneezing.

The indicated remedy may be given as a 200 C every 4 to 6 hours for 24 hours, then every 6- 8 hours for the next 24 hours, after which it should be continued every 6 - 12 hours as needed. The correct remedy should elicit a significant effect in the first 24 hours. If the patient's response to the remedy is not significant after 24 hours of frequent dosing, the remedy is incorrect and should be discontinued.

Hydrotherapy with alternating hot and cold compresses can be used to enhance circulation to the sinuses, thereby decreasing congestion, relieving pain and pressure, and facilitating healing.

Hydrotherapy Treatment for Sinusitis

Materials needed:

- 3 washcloths
- Nonabsorbent material such as wool
- 2 bowls large enough to soak washcloths
- Kettle with boiled water

1) Fill one bowl with cold water and ice.
2) Fill second bowl with water as hot as is safely tolerated. The kettle is kept handy to refresh the hot bowl as needed to keep the temperature hot.
3) Place 1 washcloth in the bowl of cold water and 2 washcloths in the hot water.
4) Wring out one hot washcloth and place over sinuses.
5) Immediately cover with a piece of wool or other insulating, nonabsorbent material and leave for 3 minutes.
6) After 3 minutes the 2nd washcloth in the hot bowl is wrung out

and placed over the sinuses to replace the first washcloth. This provides a boost of heat to prepare for the cold application.

7) The cold cloth is immediately wrung out and the second hot cloth removed and replaced with the cold which is then covered with the nonabsorbant material and left for 1 minute.
8) This process should be repeated several times with the final application always ending in cold.

This treatment is most effective if accompanied by a hot foot bath, in which the feet of the patient are placed into a tub of water as hot as is comfortably tolerated. The kettle of boiled water may be kept nearby to warm both the bowl and tub of hot water.

Needless to say it is important to have the patient remove their feet from the tub before adding the boiled water!

Anemopis californica (Yerba Mansa) Saururaceae

The fleshy roots of this plant are gathered for medicine. The leaves are also used but are said to be less strong. A 1:5 tincture prepared from fresh root or a 1:2 preparation of dried root can be dosed at 30 - 60 drops 5 times per day for acute sinusitis. When adding equal parts horseradish tincture, this dose can be doubled. For chronic conditions, 30 drops 3 to 4 times per day is often sufficient.

When using a tea, a single teaspoon of root may be decocted for each cup of water, with 1 - 4 cups per day being the usual dose.

Yerba mansa is well indicated for boggy, inflamed mucous membranes, especially when inflammation is low grade, sub-acute, or chronic and tissues are pale rather than bright red. The plant mobilizes stagnant fluids in mucous membranes, including respiratory and urinary tracts.

In the urinary tract, yerba mansa should be considered for use with cystitis or urethritis and may aid in enhancing the excretion of uric acid through the kidneys. It has anti-microbial properties with anti-fungal, anti-bacterial, anti-inflammatory, astringent, and diuretic actions. It is specifically indicated where there is stagnation of fluids and catarrh.

I have used yerba mansa primarily in the treatment of acute and chronic sinusitis. It is of interest that many cases of chronic sinusitis seen in modern practice are thought to be fungal rather than bacterial, perhaps from the habitual use of anti-biotics.

Yerba mansa has also been used for colds, pharyngitis, (here it should be gargled before swallowing), chronic otitis media, dysentery, gastritis and ulcers of stomach and duodenum. (Moore)

For mouth sores and inflammation of the gums, powdered herb can be applied topically. Powder can also be used topically to treat athlete's foot, tinea (ringworm), and diaper rash. For the latter it combines well with powdered Chilopsis (Desert Willow). Topical applications will always be helped by internal dosing of anti-fungal immune modulating herbs, such as Spilanthes, Thuja, Usnea, or others.

It is wise to be mindful of the source for this plant, as much of yerba mansa's habitat has been polluted by big business agriculture (Moore). The plant likes wetland areas and is native to much of the southwest United States.

Constituents are largely warming aromatics with some tannins.

Herbs for Cough

Acute coughs heal more quickly when herbs are dosed frequently. Sixty drops of a tincture with 6 - 8 herbs can be dosed every two hours while awake for the first 2 - 3 days, and then decreased to every 4 hours. A combination of stimulating and soothing expectorants serves to loosen mucous, ease irritation and pain in the bronchial tree, and render coughs more productive.

Herbs high in resins, such as Grindelia, Balsamorrhiza, or Eriodictyon, act as expectorants by stimulating secretions in the respiratory tract. Other more demulcent herbs, like Verbascum, Glycerrhiza, or Tussilago, facilitate expectoration by nourishing and moistening mucous membranes. A synergy results when the two types of herbs are utilized together in the same formula, each class of herb working differently to encourage a decrease in inflammation and irritation, more productive expectoration, and less spasm.

Selection of herbs is also guided by the patient presentation. Allergic coughs will respond to a different set of herbs than coughs associated with infection. The patient with asthma will need bronchodilating, antispasmodic, and anti-allergic herbs, while the persistent, exhausting cough of pertussis (whooping cough) will call for anti-spasmodic and demulcent herbs.

Adaptogens should always be included in the treatment of asthma and pertussis (whooping cough). In asthma, adaptogens aid to address underlying etiologies of allergy, as well as inflammation. In pertussis, the cough can be so exhausting, that parents and patient alike are prone to get run down from lack of sleep and worry. The inclusion of adaptogens helps maintain strength and stamina while the disease runs its course.

Althea officinalis (Marshmallow Root) Malvaceae

The powdered root of Althea can be added to juices or made into a gruel for frequent dosing. (see Chapter 7 on Digestive Function for Althea gruel recipe) Althea has strong demulcent qualities, is anti-inflammatory, mildly anti-spasmodic, moistening and nourishing to mucous membranes throughout the body.

This plant is very safe and may be dosed freely and frequently. Cut and dried root can also be used in tea, although a cold infusion will be more effective at extracting mucilage for demulcent qualities.

Ammi visnaga (Khella) Umbelliferae

Khella has both anti-allergic and anti-spasmodic activities. It is useful in formulas for asthma, as its anti-spasmodic activity is specific to the bronchial tree. It also acts as a coronary artery vasodilator and should be considered as part of a treatment plan for angina.[65] A 1:3 extract of dried seeds can be dosed at 60 drops 4 times per day. I have generally used this herb in formulas for asthma or acute coughs with a great deal of spasm, particularly if allergy is part of the underlying etiology.

Aralia spp. (Spikenard) Araliaceae

Aralia is specific for loose wet coughs and should be considered for the smokers cough or the debilitated patient with a productive cough. Aralia is discussed in more detail in the chapter on adrenal adaptogens.

Asclepias tuberosa(Pleurisy Root) Asclepidaceae

The roots of Asclepias have traditionally been used for bronchitis, pneumonia, influenza, pleurisy and pleural effusion. The plant acts in part through its powerful action as a diaphoretic, where it may be combined with ginger or cayenne for the first stage of cold or flu. A short, dry, hacking cough that is so painful the patient struggles to suppress it will likely be helped by Asclepias. The Eclectic physicians combined it with Aconitum and/or Bryonia for pleurisy. Its powerful diaphoretic actions make it a specific for patients with hot dry skin, although perspiration does not contradict its use.

In his book Plant Medicine in Practice, Dr. Bill Mitchell notes that Dr. John Bastyr used Asclepias at doses of 20 drops every 2 hours for pleural effusion, where he reported it to be reliable in reducing fluid buildup in the pleural cavity within a short period of time.[66]

Asclepias has potentially toxic cardiac glycosides that slow and strengthen the heart rate and decrease elevated blood pressure. Although toxic doses of Ascleias are likely to cause nausea and vomiting first, the plant does have potential for significant cardiotoxicity if dosed too vigorously. On the other hand these same glycosides provide the plant with the ability to improve tachycardia with ineffective cardiac output, as is seen in congestive heart failure.

The plant also contains flavonoids which undoubtedly contribute to anti-inflammatory activity.

A reasonable prescription of a 1:1 tincture of Asclepias should not exceed divided doses totaling 120 drops over a 24 hour period. As more frequent dosing works best in acute conditions, 10 - 15 drops every few hours might be more effective than 30 drops 4 times per day. When higher dosing is used for very acute conditions such as pleuritic pain, pneumonia, or pleural effusion, heart rate should be closely monitored and doses should be reduced if nausea or bradycardia occurs.

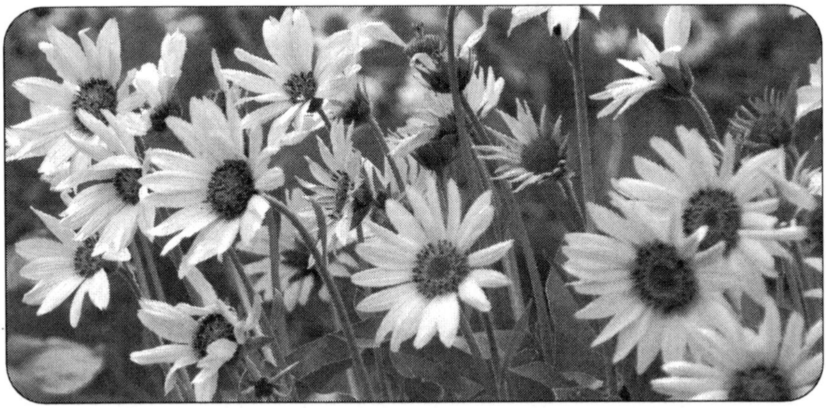

Balsam Root *Photo courtesy of Tammi Miller*

Balsamorrhiza sagitatta (Balsam Root) Compositae

The strikingly beautiful, yellow flowers of Balsamorrhiza look like low growing sunflowers, decorating dry hillsides and meadows in western states and provinces. Resins contained in the root make this a stimulating expectorant. Flavonoids and inulin are also present.

Roots should be processed quickly after being dug from the earth, as they become rock hard and nearly impossible to work with soon after harvest.

Crataegus spp. (Hawthorne) Rosaceae

Hawthorne is specifically indicated for respiratory conditions when a sensation of constriction or heaviness in the chest accompanies cough. In asthma it serves as an excellent broncho-dilator, where it acts quickly to relieve asthmatic broncho-spasm when taken at the first sign of symptoms. It can often replace inhaler use when given as a simple with instructions to take a dropperful at the first sign of broncho-spasm, repeating every minute or so as needed. It may also bring relief to patients suffering with chronic obstructive pulmonary disease (COPD). Detailed descriptions of the multiple uses for hawthorne may be read in the chapter on hawthorne.

Eriodictyon californicum (Yerba santa) Hydrophyllaceae

The sticky leaves of yerba santa are rich in resins, making it an excellent stimulating expectorant. Eriodictyon is also somewhat antimicrobial and broncho-dilating. Like most resinous expectorants, the plant's actions will be well balanced by the inclusion of demulcent herbs in the formula. Felter recommends using this herb for coughs with excessive mucous production and easy expectoration. Care should be taken that expectoration is not suppressed by the drying action of yerba santa.

Carminative actions aid in digestive function and it may be particularly useful when cough is accompanied by mild indigestion and anorexia.

Eupatorium perfoliatum (Boneset) Asteraceae

Eupatorium is specific for influenza with deep achiness in the muscles and periosteum, causing the patient to feel as if the pain of the flu has gotten into the bones. It is best used for the beginning of flu as a hot tea where it acts as an excellent diaphoretic and immune modulator. In these cases, one teaspoon of herb can be infused into each cup of hot water. If tincture is used, dosage is generally limited to no more than 40 drops 4 times per day as this herb does have potential toxicity. Fifteen drops of tincture taken 3 times per day will usually suffice as a synergist when other herbs are used.

Eclectic physicians prescribed Eupatorium for treating malaria, broncho-pneumonia, and the pain of pleurisy. (Felter) As an expectorant, Eupatorium is specific for hoarseness with an irritable or moist cough in patients too weak to produce a cough strong enough to bring about expectoration.

Eupatorium has proven useful in clinic as an intercurrent herb in the treatment of viral chronic fatigue syndrome. A tincture of 15 drops 3 - 4 times per day may be helpful when accompanied by constitutional treatment that addresses lymph and liver congestion and adrenal fatigue. A hot tea utilized in conjunction with a hydrotherapy treatment would probably be more beneficial than a tincture, however, as the tea is more likely induce diaphoresis, one of the principal healing qualities of the herb.

Eupatorium has a very strong bitter taste lending it activity as a digestive stimulant and cholagogue.

Homeopathic preparations are highly effective at relieving bone pain in fracture. A 200 C potency may be taken every 4 - 8 hours as needed, alternating with Arnica for soft tissue pain.

Long term use or overdosing of this plant can lead to liver or kidney problems, making short-term use preferable. Nausea and vomiting are generally the first signs of acute overdose.

Glycerrhiza glabra (Licorice Root) Fabaceae

Licorice is immune modulating, anti-bacterial, anti-viral, anti-inflammatory, anti-spasmodic, anti-allergic, adaptogenic, and moistening to mucous membranes, making it an excellent respiratory herb for bacterial, viral, and allergic conditions. Licorice makes a tasty addition to any respiratory tea. For more on Licorice, see the chapter on adaptogens.

Grindelia spp. (Gum Weed) Asteraceae

High in a saponin-like resin, the sticky yellow buds and flowers of Grindelia work well as a stimulating expectorant. Grindelia is specific for harsh, dry coughs with a raw sensation in the chest and soreness of pectoral muscles. (Felter) As an anti-spasmodic, it has also found use in asthma and chronic obstructive pulmonary disease as well as the spasmodic coughing of acute or subacute bronchitis.

Ligusticum porteri (Osha) Umbelliferae

Osha root, a hot spicy member of the carrot family, is known in certain parts of Native America as "Singing Herb." One woman, on first tasting the herb and knowing nothing of its properties, was seized by a sudden desire to stand up and sing. A fiery warrior of a plant, this herb can be a helpful ally in restoring courage when we lack the strength or ability to speak effectively. The plant opens the heart energy as well, reminding us to speak from our hearts rather than from the ego place of our heads especially when speaking from a fiery place.

Osha is particularly useful in viral infections affecting the respiratory tract. Although the more abundant hawthorne is a more ecologically appropriate herb for resolving acute bronchospasm, osha may be more efficacious for the overly intellectual individual struggling with asthma. In these patients, a 2 -3 inch piece of root can be carried in the shirt pocket, near the heart chakra. When symptoms of chest constriction and dyspnea threaten to come on, the patient chews on the end of the root, then holds the root to his nose and inhales deeply. The aromatic oils enter the nasal passages, drop to the bronchi, and open the airways quite quickly. It is best to reserve its use for those specific patients who do not respond to hawthorne, as it is not as common in nature as other herbs and could easily be overharvested if not used wisely.

Essential oils also lend carminative activity, helping digestion as well as respiratory complaints.

Lobaria pulmonaria (Sticta) Lichenes

Formerly called Sticta pulmonaria, this plant is a flat lichen that looks rather like one might imagine the inside lining of the lungs to appear. It prefers rainy forests and may be found in much of the Pacific Northwest.

Sticta is very specific for coughs accompanied by inflammation of nasal sinuses, with a sense of fullness and pressure in the sinuses.

A hacking cough that results in soreness of pectoral muscles is specific for Sticta, which will help relieve muscle pain as well as soothe

the cough and enhance expectoration. It has found use in spasmodic conditions of the respiratory tract including asthma, chronic obstructive pulmonary disease, and pertussis (whooping cough).

Sticta contains mucilage, giving it demulcent activity, and quercitin, suggesting it may be of use in allergic conditions of the gastrointestinal tract. The esteemed naturopathic physician, Dr. John Bastyr used Sticta for ulcerative colitis.[67]

Sticta also has anti-microbial activity.

As a tea, 1 -2 teaspoons of dried herb may be used for each cup of water. Several cups per day may be used. Some sources suggest decocting the lichen while others recommend infusion.

Tincture dosing of a 1:5 preparation of dried herb is up to 160 drops per day given in several doses throughout the day.

Lobelia inflata (Lobelia) Lobeliaceae

Lobelia is best known for its anti-spasmodic and expectorant actions in the respiratory tract. Bronchial inflammation and irritation with a spasmodic dry cough are specific indications for this herb. Lobelia is popularly used in chronic formulas for asthma and is one of the key herbs in a formula that often proves helpful in pertussis.

A 1:2 fresh plant extract can be dosed in small, but frequent divided doses to equal no more than a total of 60 drops in 24 hours. Doses in excess of this are likely to induce nausea and vomiting as Lobelia has significant emetic activity.

Lobelia is contraindicated in pneumonia, pneumothorax, hypertension, heart disease, and nervous exhaustion. Claims of toxicity are disputed as reported cases are unclear and historically influenced by anti-Thompsonian politics. (For more information on this fascinating history please refer to Medical Herbalism, Vol.10, #1 & 2, "*Is Lobelia Toxic*" by Paul Bergner). Neurological and cardiovascular symptoms including changes in level of consciousness, tremors, weakness, paralysis, tachycardia, collapse and death have been reported. Certainly a very likely effect of overdosing Lobelia might be electrolyte imbalance from hyperemesis. The plant should be used with care.

The alkaloid lobeline is the constituent thought to be primarily responsible for most of the plant's actions.

Marrubium vulgaris (Horehound) Lamiaceae

As a bitter member of the mint family, Marrubium increases the production of bile in the liver and enhances digestion. It is more specific for the respiratory system, however, and is especially helpful when hoarseness and throat irritation accompany the cough. Horehound was once a very popular ingredient in candied throat lozenges. As an expectorant the herb is particularly useful for dry coughs with a sensation of tightness in the chest. In these cases, Marrubium helps break up the mucous. Marrubium is also diaphoretic.

The dosage for a 1:1 tincture is 15 drops several times per day or a tea can be made by infusing 1 - 2 teaspoons of herb per cup of water. Whole plant in bloom is harvested for medicine.

Oplopanax horridum (Devil's Club) Araliaceae

Oplopanax is specific for bringing a dry, nagging, unproductive cough to fruition. For more information on Oplopanax please refer to the chapter on adaptogens.

Populus spp. (Poplar) Salicaceae

The resinous buds of the poplar tree act as a stimulating expectorant in the respiratory tract. The buds also have anti-inflammatory properties, probably due at least in part to the presence of salicylates. Appetite may be improved as a result of tonic and stimulating activities in the digestive tract. Antiseptic properties make it useful as a gargle in laryngitis and sore throat.

The buds may be infused and taken as a tea, but as resins do not extract well in water, an alcoholic extract may be preferable. A 1:3 tincture can be dosed at 10 to 15 drops every 2 hours or 30 drops 4 times daily.

Prunus spp. (Wild Cherry Bark) Rosaceae

Like most members of the rose family, Prunus is abundant in tannins, giving it astringent properties. The presence of plant resins makes it a stimulating expectorant. Prunus is particularly good when the cough is accompanied by digestive weakness. It acts as a nutritive tonic, carminative, and digestive stimulant. The roots are soothing to irritated, inflamed mucous membranes and the plant is generally calming to the nervous system.

Prunus does contain a cyanogenic glycoside, which is highest in the seeds and possibly wilted leaves. It is best to use only the bark, stick to recommended doses, and avoid prolonged use.

Teas can be decocted with 1 teaspoon of dried bark per cup of water or a 1:3.5 tincture can be dosed at 20 drops every 2 hours for up to 8 doses or 40 drops 4 times per day.

Thymus vulgaris (Thyme) Lamiaceae

The leaves and flowers of the common garden thyme used in cooking provide excellent anti-spasmodic, bronchodilating, and expectorant activities in the respiratory tract. The herb also has some anti-fungal and anti-bacterial activity, at least in part due to the presence of essential oils. Disinfectant qualities of the essential oils make thyme a great addition to inhale in a steam treatment. Typical tincture doses are 30 drops 3 - 4 times daily. A teaspoon of leaves can be infused into a cup of water for use as a tea.

Trifolium pratense (Red Clover) Fabaceae

Like many members of the pea family, red clover contains isoflavones that are hormone modulating, making it a useful plant for patients with reproductive hormone imbalances. As an alterative, red clover blossoms are used for chronic skin conditions and cancer. Trifolium also acts to facilitate lymphatic circulation. Dr. Bill Mitchell used it especially for cancers involving the lymph system.[68]

In respiratory conditions, expectorant, anti-bacterial, and anti-spasmodic actions add to its alterative properties. It soothes inflammation, dry irritated mucous membranes, and pharyngitis. Coughs may be unproductive, spasmodic, and possibly even explosive in nature.

The exhausting, violently spasmodic cough of pertussis (whooping cough) may be aided by the addition of red clover blossoms. It has also been used for patients recovering from flu or other acute respiratory states.

The addition of Trifolium to a respiratory formula adds what the old books call blood cleansing properties, which is simply a way of suggesting that a plant has the ability to reduce the toxic load in the blood. Often, this is done either by enhancing the function of detoxification and excretory organs or by improving blood and lymph circulation.

The pretty colored flowers add color as well as medicine to any respiratory tea prescription. As a single herb in a tea, one tablespoon of red clover can be infused per cup of water and 4 cups taken per day. Tincture can be given at doses of 15 to 60 drops up to four times per day.

Tussilago farfara (Eastern Coltsfoot) Asteraceae

Due to the presence of hepatotoxic pyrrolizidine alkaloids, Tussilago is best reserved for short-term use, and should be avoided in patients with compromised liver function or known difficulty with phase two detoxification pathways. Although it has traditionally been used for chronic conditions, environmental pollutants have overtaxed hepatic detoxification pathways, making it increasingly difficult for our bodies to process these alkaloids.

Both Petasites (western coltsfoot) and Tussilago put their flowers up in spring, with leaves appearing only after the flowers. Both herbs may be used as anti-spasmodics, expectorants, and demulcents for respiratory conditions but both also contain pyrrolizidine alkaloids. The yellow flowers of Tussilago bloom perky and bright about three inches from the ground while the green leaves sprout up later, soft and demulcent.

Both flowers and leaves may be used for medicine. Traditionally 1 - 2 teaspoons of herb was infused into each cup of water, with several (4 - 6) cups taken throughout the day. I generally use this herb as a supportive demulcent in a formula blended for tea. Tincture may be administered in divided doses throughout the day for a total of 120 drops in 24 hours, but again I generally stick to lower doses and use it in formula.

Verbascum thapsus (Mullein) Scrophulariaceae

Acting as both a stimulating and soothing expectorant, Verbascum, is a valuable addition to any respiratory formula. The plant also has anti-spasmodic activity, making it useful for asthma and spasmodic conditions of the intestinal tract. Both flowers and leaves may be used for medicine with flowers adding sedative properties to calm frayed nerves.

Summary of Actions of Respiratory Herbs

Soothing Demulcent Expectorants

Demulcents will be anti-inflammatory through their ability to soothe, nourish and rebuild mucous membrane surfaces.

Altheaofficinalis (Marshmallow Root)
Glycerrhiza glabra (Licorice Root)
Petasites spp. (Western Coltsfoot)
Lobaria pulmonaria (Sticta)
Tussilago farfara (Eastern Coltsfoot)
Verbascum Thapsus (Mullein)

Expectorants

Ascelpias tuberosa (Pleurisy Root)
Balsamorrhiza sagitatta (Balsam Root)
Eriodictyon californicum (California Poppy)
Eupatorium perfoliatum (Boneset)
Grindelia spp. (Gumweed)
Ligusticum porteri (Osha)
Lobelia inflata (Lobelia)
Marrubium vulgaris (Horehound)
Oplopanax horridum (Devil's Club)
Prunus spp. (Wild Cherry Bark)
Lobaria pulmonaria (Sticta)
Thymus vulgaris (Garden Thyme)
Verbascum thapsus (Mullein)

Anti-Inflammatory

Asclepias tuberosa (Pleurisy Root)
Balsamorrhiza sagitatta (Balsam Root) Flavonoids
Crataegus spp. (Hawthorne) Flavonoids
Glycerrhiza glabra (Licorice Root) Adrenal & Demulcent
Populus spp. (Poplar Buds)
Prunus spp. (Wild Cherry Bark)
Lobaria pulmonaria (Sticta)
Trifolium pretense (Red Clover)

Anti-Spasmodics

Ammi visnaga (Khella)
Crataegus spp. (Hawthorne)
Glycerhiza glabra (Licorice Root)
Grindelia spp. (Gumweed)
Ligusticum porteri (Osha)
Lobelia inflata (Lobelia)
Petasites (Western Coltsfoot)
Thymus vulgaris (Garden Thyme)
Trifolium pratense (Red Clover)
Tussilago farfara (Eastern Coltsfoot)
Verbascum

Anti-Allergic

Ammi visnaga (Khella)
Crataegus spp. (Hawthorne)
Ephedra sinensis (Chhinese Ephedra)
Glycerrhiza glabra (Licorice Root)
Lobaria pulmonaria (Sticta) Quercitin

Anti-Microbial

Eupatorium perfoliatum (Boneset)
Glycerrhiza glabra (Licorice Root)
Ligusticum porter (Osha)
Lobaria pulmonaria (Sticta)
Thymus vulgaris (Garden Thyme)
Trifolium pretense (Red Clover)

Antiseptic

Populus spp. (Popular Buds)

Digestive

Crataegus spp. (Hawthorne)
Eupatorium perfoliatum (Boneset)
Ligusticum porter (Osha)
Marrbium vulgaris (Horehound)
Petasites (Western Coltsfoot)Populus spp. (Poplar Buds)
Prunus spp. (Wild Cherry Bark)
Thymus vulgaris (Garden Thyme)

Prescribing Formulas for Coughs

The ideal cough formula will vary with the symptom presentation of the patient and the condition being treated. Selecting herbs based on specific indications often leads to better results, but sometimes the best formula is made with the herbs at hand.

Generally a mix of resinous and demulcent expectorants with an immune modulating herb creates a foundation for a good cough formula. Anti-spasmodic or anti-asthmatic herbs can be added in as indicated.

For optimal results in treating acute conditions, a formula of 6 - 8 herbs can be dosed every two hours for a couple days then every four hours until symptoms have resolved.

Pertussis/Whooping Cough

The number of pertussis cases that are diagnosed and reported has been increasing since the 1980's. As a result of the rising number of actual cases, health care practitioners have become more alert to the possibility that a lingering, exhaustive, spasmodic, cough may be pertussis. This increased awareness leads to more testing, diagnosis, and subsequent reporting of the disease. In addition, many parents are electing not to immunize their children, and although it has been obvious to me, in my own practice, that pertussis epidemics are more prevalent in non-immunized groups of children in the community, noncompliance with vaccine recommendations is only one player in the return of the disease.[69]

The newer acellular vaccine, DTaP, appears to be less effective for long term immunity than the previous whole cell vaccine, DPT. The change from whole cell to acellular vaccines was instituted in the 1990's in response to international concerns about side effects, including rare, but serious, permanent neurological damage in children who had just received the vaccine. Whole cell vaccines were also commonly associated with fever, and pain and swelling at the injection site.[70]

The wracking, intensely spasmodic cough that is typical of pertussis generally develops a week or two after initial flu like symptoms and may persist for a few weeks more. The typical violently spasmodic cough, which is often worse at night, disturbs sleep, and can be exhausting to parents and children alike. While most children recover, infants and elderly folks who contract pertussis are more prone to develop pneumonia, and there are a certain number of infants that are lost each year as a result of pertussis.

Because infants do not have immune systems that are developed enough to respond to a vaccine, immunization of newborns, with either the old DTP or the newer DTaP, is not effective as a preventive measure. Immunization of adults and older children whose immune systems are mature enough to mount an immune response has been done to prevent the disease and consequent exposure of more vulnerable populations. However, it appears that more frequent boosters with DTaP are required to maintain this immunity. In addition, there is no guarantee that individuals who are immunized will not contract the disease, if they are exposed, although the disease tends to be less severe in these cases.

Nosodes, which are homeopathic medicines made from diseased tissue, have been used in epidemics throughout the history of homeopathy, with generally good success. My experience with Influenzinum for prevention of flu has been so gratifying, (see section on influenza) that my faith in nosodes has grown tremendously.

For those parents who do not elect to immunize their children against pertussis, I generally recommend Pertussinum 200 C to be taken each fall, a few pellets once each week for three weeks, to be repeated again once or twice per week if exposure to pertussis occurs or if cases begin showing up in the community. In epidemics, which usually occur in cycles of every 3 - 5 years, I dispense Pertussinum 30 C or 200 C as a booster for immunized patients as well as nonimmunized patients, in hopes of boosting the immunity conferred by the vaccines.

Whether parents decide to immunize their children or not, it is important that we consider the health of our whole community, and not just ourselves and our own families. Certainly, at the very least, infants and elders should not be unnecessarily exposed to any one, child or adult, who is suffering with an upper respiratory infection.

Patients affected by pertussis will do best if they are treated for a year after recovery from the acute infection, as pertussis often leaves the lungs and bronchi vulnerable. Verbascum, glycerrhiza, althea, trifolium, aralia and oplopanax are some of the nourishing, rebuilding herbs that should be considered for restoration of optimal health after an episode of pertussis.

Herbs to consider in formulas for treating acute pertussis include lobelia, verbascum, glycerrhiza, grindelia, althea, and thyme. These herbs have proven highly effective at mitigating symptoms, allowing everyone more rest, and preventing complications. Parents and affected children should all be treated with adrenal adaptogens during the child's illness to prevent exhaustion, Glycerrhiza being the adaptogen of choice for the affected child.

Many of the old homeopathic texts suggest using homeopathic Drosera for the treatment of pertussis. While this remedy has certainly proven helpful in reducing symptoms, it has not been as helpful as the herbs in this author's experience. Often another remedy is needed, and in many cases remedies seem to help for a few days then stop working and another remedy must be used.

Use of the nosode Pertussinum in a 30C or 200C potency may help other therapies work more effectively and should be used to prevent other family members or exposed individuals from contracting the disease. The nosode can be given once per day for three days, then every 3 - 7 days for as long as exposure continues. The same dose can be given to the infected child.

Asthma/Chronic Obstructive Pulmonary Disease (COPD)

Symptoms of asthma usually manifest as a result of a hypersensitivity response to external stimuli. For some patients, asthma can be a component of seasonal allergies or hay fever, with episodes triggered by pollens or grasses. Symptoms may also be triggered by molds or chemical toxins. These patients will generally do well with nutritional and herbal support of liver function and detoxification pathways, in addition to anti-allergic and anti-asthma protocols.

Most patients with acute or chronic respiratory disease will find that their symptoms are aggravated by the ingestion of milk and milk containing foods. Some patients may have other food sensitivities as well, with wheat and gluten being top offenders. Avoidance of offending substances is important in reducing symptoms of asthma.

Adrenal support is crucial to address allergic and inflammatory mechanisms at play in asthma, as well as improve stamina and emotional well being. While any of the adrenal adaptogens may be of service, Glycerrhiza glabra, Aralia spp., Uncaria tomentosa, Ocimum sanctum, and Ganoderma lucidum are more specifically indicated for the treatment of asthma. Vitamin C and B complex are also important, with vitamin B-5 being specifically beneficial in supporting adrenal function.

Flavonoid rich herbs will also help allay inflammation and hypersensitivity reactions. Hawthorne, rose hips, and dark purple to deep red colored berries are full of particularly helpful anthocyanidin type flavonoids. Many of these berries can be included in the diet. The rose hips jam, described in the section on hay fever, is a tasty way to increase flavonoid intake and reduce hypersensitivity reactions.

Herbal prescriptions should include plants that are anti-spasmodic, anti-allergic, broncho-dilating, and demulcent. In addition to a formula of herbs that includes all these properties, another prescription is advised for use in acute flare-ups.

As described in the chapter on hawthorne, 30 drops of a tincture of hawthorne can be taken as often as needed for acute broncho-spasm. Acute symptoms of dyspnea (difficulty breathing) will often be relieved within 3- 5 doses. Hawthorne has also been of help in relieving acute breathing difficulties for patients with emphysema and other types of COPD.

In cases where hawthorne does not prove to be of service, a 2- 3 inch piece of osha root (Ligusticum porteri) may be carried in the pocket and used as described in the section on Ligusticum. Because osha is less abundant in nature, it is best to start with hawthorne.

Although Ephedra sinensis (Chinese ephedra) is a very effective anti-allergic bronchodilator, it is also very stimulating and can produce the same side effects of restlessness, anxiety, and agitation that many patients experience with pharmaceutical inhalers used to reduce broncho-spasm. Since asthmatic patients tend to be more sensitive, they are the very patients more likely to experience these undesirable side effects. For this reason, the use of Ephedra sinensis should be reserved for cases in which other therapies are not proving efficacious. Not all patients will manifest symptoms of overstimulation with the use of Ephedra.

Inhalation of essential or volatile oils can also be helpful in treating acute broncho-spasm. Because the extraction of essential oils requires a large amount of plant material to produce relatively small amounts of oil, it is not necessarily the most ecologically responsible use of our herbs. In addition, essential oils are strong and most of them need to be used with caution. However, that having been said, essential oils have an important place in herbal prescribing.

Essential oils of eucalyptus, peppermint, and thyme may all be inhaled to alleviate symptoms of acute broncho-spasm. The oils are anti-microbial as well as broncho-dilating. Although Eucalyptus is particularly popular, my personal favorite is peppermint oil.

A few drops of the essential oil can be mixed into hot water and used as a steam inhalation. When Osha root is used for inhalation, it is the essential oils in the plant that we rely on for alleviation of acute broncho-spasm.

Case: Where Diagnosis Made the Difference

The following case illustrates the importance of selecting herbs that address the underlying etiology of a cough. It also offers a few examples of formulating for both infectious and allergic respiratory conditions.

A 47 year old woman came to the clinic complaining of a cough that had been going on for 3 weeks. She reported a history of pneumonia two years earlier, which had been treated with anti-biotics. Her cough was mostly loose, with easy expectoration at some times and more difficult at others. She felt a "wheezy, rattling, and rumbling" in her chest and a sensation of constriction. The cough was sometimes spasmodic, occasionally waking her at night. She also reported some coryza with a plugged sensation in her nose and ears. She had mild myalgia in the muscles of her back which she attributed to the coughing. Despite these symptoms, her energy remained fairly good. She was able to go to work and felt only slightly more fatigued than usual.

On auscultation, (listening to the patient's lungs with a stethoscope) her right lower to middle lung fields were wheezy and wet sounding, though lung sounds were not diminished and no obvious rales (a particular type of sound that can be heard in some types of lung congestion) were appreciated. Examination of her ears revealed mild serous effusion (fluid). Her tonsils were slightly enlarged but there was an absence of redness in her throat. Cervical lymph nodes were also mildly enlarged.

Suspecting possible mycoplasma pneumonia, (walking pneumonia) the appropriate lab work (Complete Blood Count/CBC with manual differential and cold agglutinins) was ordered and the patient was sent for a chest X-ray. Spinal manipulation to her cervical and thoracic spine was performed to ensure optimal innervation to the respiratory organs and to relieve stress on the musculo-skeletal system precipitated by three weeks of hard coughing.

Because I was worried about an infectious respiratory condition, and possible pneumonia, I prescribed the following aggressive treatment plan:

A tincture:

Ligusticum porteri (Osha root).........2 drams
Grindelia spp. (Gum Weed) ....2 drams
Lobaria pulmonaria (Sticta) ....1 dram
Verbascum thapsus (Mullein) ....1 dram
Inula helenium (Elecampane) ....1 dram
Prunus spp. (Wild Cherry Bark) ......1 dram
DOSE: 1 teaspoon every 2 hours while awake

A tea of equal parts of:

Verbascum
Glycerrhiza
Trifolium
Tussilago farfara (Eastern Coltsfoot)
Eriodictyon californicum (Yerba Santa)
DOSE: 1 tablespoon per cup, at least 4 cups per day, more as desired

Optibiotics, a product from the Eclectic Institute in Sandy, Oregon, containing in 2 tablets:

Echinacea ....455 mg.
Allium sativa (garlic) ....195 mg.
Commiphora myrrh (Myrrh) ....190 mg.
Zingiber officianalis (Ginger) ....97 mg.
Capsicum frutescens (Cayenne) ....65mg.
Vitamin A ....10,000 I.U.
Vitamin C ....500 mg.
Vitamin B6 ....15mg.
Magnesium ....15mg.
Zinc ....15 mg.
Bioflavonoids ....500 mg.
DOSE: 2 tablets every two hours while awake

In addition to the Vitamin C in the formula she was to take 1000 mg Vitamin C every 2 hours while awake.

The patient was also instructed to apply a mustard plaster to her chest for 20 minutes once or twice daily.

Despite this aggressive treatment regimen, the patient reported that she was really not much better on follow up 24 hours later. Although her cough was slightly more productive, the change was minimal and she was no better in any other way. This is unusual, as herbal cough formulas invariably bring easier expectoration and relief from symptoms even when they do not act curatively alone.

By this time the results of the chest X-ray were back, reporting "findings most consistent with pneumonitis." Cold agglutinins blood work was negative for mycoplasma and differential white blood cell count/WBC was unremarkable for either bacterial or viral infection.

Since pneumonitis is often a hypersensitivity (allergic) reaction and blood work was negative for significant infection, she was started on a tincture that addressed the allergic aspect of the condition:

Glycerrhiza glabra (Licorice Root) . . .1 dram
Urtica dioica (Nettles Leaf) . . . . .2 drams
Rosa spp. (Rose Hips) . . . . .2 drams
Crataegus spp. (Hawthorne) . . . . .1 dram
Ammi visnaga (Khella) . . . . .2 drams

DOSE: 1 teaspoon every 4 hours while awake

Quercitin, an anti-allergic flavonoid that naturally occurs in onions, was also given at a dose of 500 mg. three times per day.

Since she already had the formulas at hand, the Optibiotic was reduced to 2 capsules 4 times per day to retain the positive effects of the Vitamin A on mucous membrane health and nourish the immune system, thereby preventing possible secondary infection. The original tincture was continued at 60 drops (1/2 teaspoon) four times per day for respiratory support and as an expectorant, and the tea was continued at one teaspoon per cup twice per day and as desired.

On follow up 48 hours later, the patient reported a dramatic change. The congestion in both the lungs and sinuses had cleared considerably, her ears were no longer plugged, her energy was back and her sleep was no longer disturbed by the cough. The anti-allergic properties of the herbs in the second formula were more capable of directly addressing the underlying pathology of the respiratory symptoms.

Influenza

Flu has a habit of really making press every few years, and while it is sometimes difficult to distinguish hysterical fear from a true need for concern in the face of a predicted flu epidemic, prevention is surely the best way to go, although not necessarily through potentially immune-suppressive vaccination. There are other highly effective and much safer options for enhancing immune health and preventing flu.

Needless to say, optimal diet, fresh air, and keeping channels of elimination open are just as essential for prevention of flu as in any other situation. With that basic foundation set in place, the addition of a homeopathic nosode, Influenzinum, has proven highly efficacious in clinic at preventing flu. The first year I used it for all my patients, none of them came down with the flu and the only flu cases I saw in the office that year were new patients. No one was more astonished than the prescribing physician!

Influenzinum 30C can be given once a day for 3 days for 3 weeks in the fall, and repeated once per month during flu season. Extra doses can be added every 4 hours as needed for the first sign of flu or once or twice a day for 3 - 4 days if exposure has occurred. Patients who took the nosode at the first sign of flu were able to successfully ward off further symptoms. On a rare occasion, patients will still get the flu, but generally these patients are very run down or already well into their symptoms by the time they take the Influenzinum.

The berries of Sambucus nigra (elderberry) are fine medicine for warding off symptoms when taken at the first sign of flu. This herb, high in anthocyanidin type flavonoids, addresses vulnerable terrain by acting as an anti-oxidant, anti-inflammatory, and immune modulator. Elderberry can be taken in small doses throughout the winter to prevent, as well as treat, flu. Combining berries with elder flowers adds a calming quality to the medicine.

Garlic is an excellent medicine for use in prevention and treatment of flu. A quarter teaspoon of the garlic vinegar described in the chapter on hypertension can be taken once per day for prevention, increased to 4 times per day if symptoms occur.

If, despite all this excellent care, we are struck down by an infection with flu virus, it helps to remember that such illnesses do offer the body an opportunity to clean house. The detoxification process can be aided by hydrotherapy such as sweating and fever treatments, constitutional hydrotherapy treatments, or warming sheet packs. Warming tee shirt treatments or mustard plasters can help increase circulation to the lungs, while the application of warming socks at bedtime helps pull congestion from the head.

The correct homeopathic remedy is an invaluable ally in these cases, and although the process can sometimes be disheartening as there are so many remedies to choose from, the results of prescribing the right remedy are well worth the effort. The action of the specific remedy for the case is enhanced when the nosode, Influenzinum, is continued along with it.

Although I have mixed a wide variety of herbal formulas for all the patients I have treated over the years with flu, in the end, I find a simple kitchen remedy is really the best. A teaspoon or so of lemon juice, 2 - 3 cloves of raw chopped garlic and a pinch of cayenne or a half teaspoon of grated fresh ginger are mixed together in a quart jar. Boiling water is then poured over the whole concoction and the tea is taken hot. Honey can be added for its own medicine as well as to improve the taste, but some patients may need to avoid this last ingredient if blood sugar levels tend to fluctuate.

In recent years I have added elderberry syrup to the mix with good results. This simple treatment has replaced my usual respiratory tinctures and teas in recent years, as it is so simple and efficacious. Other respiratory and immune herbs can be added into the mix as well, however.

Hydrotherapy for Flu and Colds

Home Sweating Treatment

This treatment works well whenever sweating is desired for detoxification and is an excellent alternative when a sauna is not so easily available. When done at the very first sign of symptoms, a good sweat will often completely ward off a developing flu or cold. Although there are many ways to do this treatment, the following is a method that has worked well for my patients through the years.

1) Place two sheets on a comfortable rug on the floor in a warm room. (If this treatment is done on the bed there is a chance that the patient will sweat so much that the mattress may get wet) Place a pillow at the head and a hot water bottle (if available) at the feet. Cover these sheets with several warm blankets.

2) Place sweat pants, sweat shirt, and a pair of wool or other insulating socks near the bathtub.
3) Fill the tub with water as hot as can be safely tolerated.
4) Add 1 - 2 cups Epsom salts to bath if available.
5) Get into bath and cover as much of the body in hot water as possible. Remain in the bath until sweat begins to pour from the head.
6) Quickly get out of the bath, towel off, and put sweat clothes and socks on. Get between the sheets and under the blankets and remain there for twenty minutes.
7) Finish with a cold shower of 1 -2 minutes duration. Towel off, put on warm bedclothes, and go to bed for the night.
8) This treatment can be preceded by a cup of hot yarrow or ginger tea to increase benefit. It is important to stay well hydrated whenever a sweating treatment is done.

If a sauna is available, alternate back and forth between the hot sauna and a cold shower a few times, always ending in cold.

Warming Tee Shirt

This treatment encourages circulation to the lungs. It is very important that the patient is warm before doing this treatment. A cotton tee shirt is dipped in cold water and wrung out well. It may be placed in the refrigerator to keep it cool. Then a hot bath or shower may be taken to warm the patient. Once out of the warming treatment, the patient puts the tee shirt on and covers that with a shirt of non-absorbent material and goes to bed. This treatment can be combined with warming socks to obtain optimal benefit. (See end of chapter on Nervines for information on warming socks.)

Mustard Plaster

This is an old home remedy that almost never fails for relieving bronchitis, pneumonia, and chest congestion.

1) A thin cotton cloth twice the size of the patient's chest is laid out on a warmed cookie sheet, in preparation for the mustard mixture.
2) For adults, one tablespoon of good quality, medicinal grade mustard (or ginger) powder is placed in a bowl and mixed with

four tablespoons of wheat flour or ground flax seed. This should be stirred well so that the mustard is evenly dispersed.

3) Enough warm water is stirred in to make a paste.
4) The mixture is spread over half of the cotton material. The cloth is then folded in half to make a sandwich.
5) Rub olive oil onto the patient's chest, and then apply the plaster. Cover the patient well and leave for twenty minutes. (For large breasted women it may be more effective to apply the plaster to the back.)
6) If the patient experiences burning, the plaster should be removed sooner.
7) For children, increase the amount of flour or flax seed to 8 tablespoons for every one tablespoon of mustard seed powder and for infants this amount is further increased to twelve tablespoons flour or flax to each tablespoon of mustard or ginger powder.
8) The patient should be kept warm throughout the treatment and afterwards.
9) Young children and especially infants should be checked frequently and the pack should be removed if redness of the skin occurs. The skin of infants is sensitive and more prone to burning, although the diluted mixture should prevent this.
10) If a mustard or ginger plaster is needed and there is herb available that is old or not of medicinal grade quality, it will be better to use what is at hand then to do nothing, and often the treatment will still have benefit.

Constitutional hydrotherapy and wet sheet packs are more specialized, highly efficacious treatments that are utilized by naturopathic physicians.[71]

Cytokine Storm

In 2009, with the prediction of a possible deadly "swine flu" (H1N1) epidemic, concerns were raised about using so-called "immune stimulating" herbs for the treatment of influenza symptoms, due to theoretical possibilities of an overactive immune response to the virus, causing what is termed cytokine storm. It has been theorized that the large numbers of young, vital, and previously healthy patients who died during the serious 1918 influenza epidemic succumbed as a result of cytokine storm. Due to the makeup of the

H1N1 virus, it was thought that the risk of cytokine storm in young healthy people who developed flu from H1N1 could well be significant.

Symptoms of cytokine storm, due largely to overactivation of immune system cytokines, TNF alpha and IL-6 (interleukin-6), include high fever, respiratory distress, sepsis, and major organ failure. For this reason, there has been some concern among herbalists about using herbs that could be immune stimulating.

Echinacea

Although empirically safe and effective in the usual flu epidemics, Echinacea probably has the strongest reputation as an herb to be avoided during the H1N1 season. This is partly due to its reputation as an immune stimulant and partly due to research that suggests that Echinacea stimulates the very cytokines that we wanted to tone down in H1N1, namely IL-6 and TNF alpha.[72] Whether the use of Echinacea was actually of concern during that particular epidemic is still controversial, but with so many other herbs to choose from, why take chances?

It is of interest that traditional use of Echinacea (E. angustifolia) by Eclectics, who learned the medicine from Native Americans, was for sepsis, gangrenous wounds, "bad blood," typhoid, puerperal fever, and the bites of venomous snakes and insects. It was also used for chronic bronchial catarrh as well as "common nasal and bronchial catarrhs" (Felter P. 330). The plant has been shown to be anti-fungal, anti-bacterial, anti-viral, and anti-inflammatory.[73,74,75]

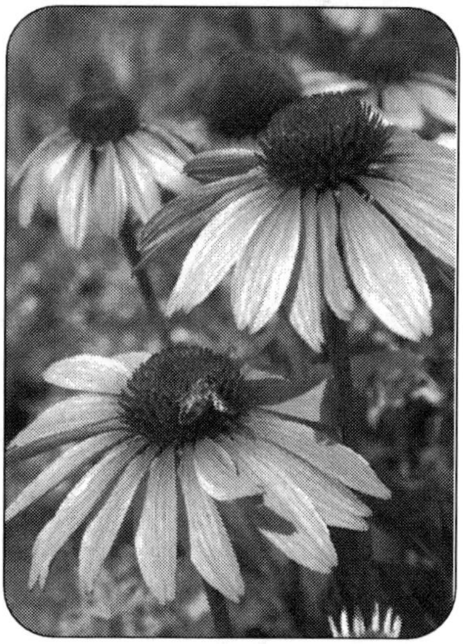

Echinacea
Photo Courtesy of Orna Izakson, N.D.

Much controversy surrounds Echinacea with concerns about its use for autoimmune disease and AIDS as well as cytokine storm. In actuality, while many practitioners use Echinacea quite successfully without adverse events in both AIDS and autoimmune patients, other practitioners report worsening of symptoms in some serious autoimmune conditions. Due to research which has focused largely on the immune stimulating properties of Echinacea, this plant has come to be seen primarily as an immune stimulant, which ignores other aspects of the plant's actions, such as blood cleansing and lymphatic properties. In any case, Echinacea is still totally safe and often efficacious for prevention and treatment for the usual winter colds and flu. The concerns surrounding the H1N1 flu are specific to that type of virus.

Echinacea has proven highly useful in clinic for infected wounds, cellulitis, abscesses, patients who have a tendency to suppuration, and in acne. It has also been useful for some cases of interstitial cystitis where it may help prevent and treat flare-ups. In all these cases it combines well with Baptisia.

There is a common misconception that Echinacea loses its efficacy if used long term. The evidence for this is very poor, and traditional and clinical uses simply do not bear this out.

Echinacea is nontoxic and may be administered often in fairly high doses for acute conditions (thirty to sixty drops of tincture every two hours) without adverse effects. For suppurative or septic conditions, its actions are potentized by the addition of Baptisia.

Hay Fever

Seasonal allergies respond well to a combination of dried nettles leaf and rose hips. Rose hips can be dispensed either as jam (see recipe below) or solid extract. The freeze dried capsules of nettle seem to work better than tincture, although tincture will certainly help. Two or three capsules of the nettles leaf should be given three to four times daily. A solid extract of rose hips is highly concentrated and can be given _ teaspoon 2 - 4 times per day. Other herbs to consider include Euphrasia and Ambrosia. A formula of adrenal adaptogens is also essential.

Urtica dioica (Nettles)

There are a number of homeopathic remedies that are useful when hay fever symptoms are more severe. The remedy will do its best work when constitutional prescribing has been started and the herbs are included as part of the treatment plan.

Wyethia has been a common remedy in clinic for the treatment of seasonal allergies, although it is by no means the only one to consider. It is mentioned here as it is a little known remedy, but common for hay fever. Guiding symptoms for the use of Wyethia include itchiness in the palate or posterior pharynx.

Patients needing Euphrasia, another common remedy for seasonal allergies, will complain of acrid lachrymation (watery eyes with irritation) accompanied by bland watery discharge from the nose (coryza). Both discharges will likely be profuse. Euphrasia is also a remedy to consider for allergic conjunctivitis. I have not seen it be effective in the more infectious conjunctivitis often seen in children. Here Pulsatilla proves to be the better choice.

Allium cepa should be considered if lachrymation is bland but coryza is acrid. Like Euphrasia, discharges will be profuse.

Most patients do well with the herbs and will not require homeopathic prescribing.

Rose Hips Jam

1) Place dried or fresh deseeded rose hips into a glass jar.
2) Cover with organic pomegranate, grape, or blueberry juice to 1/4 to 1/2 inch above the rose hips. A small part, perhaps 1/8 part, of the juice may be substituted with orange juice for extra flavor.
3) Stir in some freshly ground organic orange peel.
4) Add spices such as cinnamon or cloves as desired.
5) Leave overnight in the refrigerator. The naturally occurring pectin in the rose hips will set up overnight to make a nice jam. The jam will keep for several days in the refrigerator.

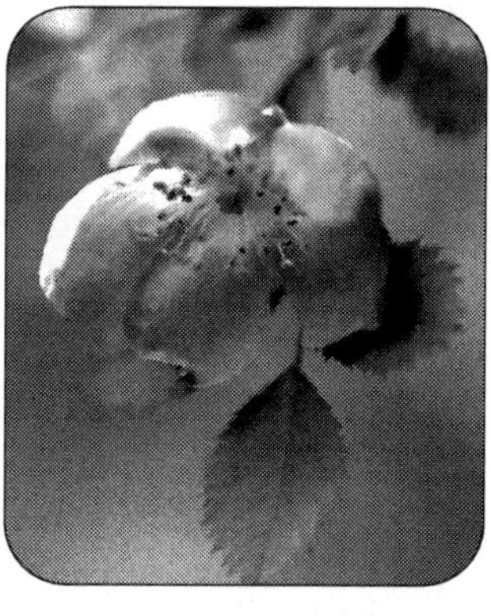

Wild Rose
Photo courtesy of Tammi Miller

For seasonal allergies, 1/2 to 1 teaspoon may be taken 4 times per day or more often.

Although other juices can be used, the anthocyanidin flavonoids in the dark colored juices add extra medicinal value to the preparation.

Variation on Rose Hips Jam

1) Simmer fresh or dried black elderberries (Sambucus nigra) in juice, preferably one of the juices mentioned above.
2) Strain to remove seeds.
3) Pour into a glass jar containing rose hips, covering rose hips by 1/4 to 1/2 inch.
4) Add spices such as cinnamon or cloves as desired.
5) Leave overnight in refrigerator. The addition of the elderberry creates an excellent flu and cold remedy.

Ceasing Cigarettes

The use of tobacco was traditionally reserved by Native Americans for prayer and ceremony. A strong, highly addictive plant, tobacco is what traditionalists might term a "power plant." Such plants are meant to be used judiciously and usually only in ceremony. Power plants used unwisely will eventually "bite back" or "steal" the personal power of the individual misusing them. In the case of tobacco, this bite can manifest with chronic, and eventually irreversible respiratory disease, as well as a host of other physical problems. Because of the strong spirit or nature of the plant, it can overpower the spirit of the smoker resulting in addiction. In these cases, the pull of the plant has more power than the will of the person to stay away from the herb.

The purpose or Medicine of tobacco is to connect us to Spirit. It is also considered to be spiritually protective, where it may help in protecting from negative influences. Such influences might include strong projections or negative emotions directed at us from another person or from a negative environment or circumstance. It is important to recognize that the smoker is filling some need with the regular use of tobacco. Meeting that need in some healthier way respects the patient's process and facilitates deeper transformation as well as aid in stopping cigarettes permanently.

When patients smoke, the first thing I suggest they do is change to a brand of cigarettes such as American Spirit that does not contain toxic chemicals and pesticides. Next I suggest they pray with each cigarette. If they are willing, I have them hand roll each cigarette, mixing in some lavender and mullein with the tobacco. The mullein is added for demulcent protection to the lungs while the lavender serves to calm the nerves and ease the transition away from tobacco.

Once the patient is willing to quit, a tincture can be used to take as needed for withdrawal symptoms. The following formula provides a basic foundation that may vary depending on individual needs. I ask patients what their symptoms have been when they have tried to quit in the past and add other flower essences accordingly. The formula is dosed at 2 - 5 drops as often as needed for symptoms of withdrawal, which usually consist of irritability or anxiety.

Piper methysticum .... 3 parts
Passiflora incarnate .... 2 parts
Lobelia inflata .... 1 part
Glycerrhiza glabra .... 2 parts
Tobacco flower essence .... 2 drops per ounce
Other flower essences as indicated

In addition a vial of homeopathic Caladium 6C, 12C, or more rarely 30C may be taken as needed for cigarette cravings.

Withdrawal will go more quickly when patients include a sweating treatment to eliminate nicotine from their system. The old writers in the naturopathic literature tell us that when cold wet sheet packs, an old treatment used to induce sweating, are used with patients withdrawing from tobacco, the sweat from the patient stains the sheets brown.

It is easy to be critical of smokers but in reality, it is not easy to stop cigarettes. Compassionate encouragement without critical nagging, combined with reframing the habit while the patient is still engaged in smoking brings in a healing energy that is much more likely to facilitate quitting than judgmental attitudes, which the smoker is very likely getting from every corner in any case.

Nasal Polyps

Nasal polyps generally respond well to a homeopathic preparation of Teucrium 30C four times per day. Constitutional treatment should also be initiated to address underlying susceptibilities.

Chapter 10
First Aid

Arnica montana

THE HOMEOPATHIC PREPARATION of this plant is a must for every first aid kit. A few pellets of the remedy taken internally as soon as possible after an injury accelerates healing and prevents swelling, pain, and bruising by mobilizing the rush of blood and lymph from the affected area, preventing stagnation and allowing for better circulation and more efficient healing. Arnica generally does its best work when given in the first 24 - 48 hours after an acute injury, the sooner the better.

A 200C potency may be given every 4 to 6 hours for the first twenty four hours after an injury. The frequency of dosing will depend somewhat on what the symptoms call for. In more severe injuries, higher potencies, such as 1M, 10M or even 50M may be given, as a one time or repeated dose. Depending upon the severity of the injury, this one time dose might be followed with a 200C or 1M every 4 to 8 hours as needed.

The exact number of pellets given is not critical, as the dosage has already been determined by the preparation into a 30C, 200C, or 1M. The remedy should be continued every 6 to 8 hours for a couple more days as needed to keep bruising, swelling, and pain to a minimum.

While I generally use this plant in its homeopathic form, it can be used herbally instead. It is a strong and potentially toxic plant, however, and should be dosed judiciously. Doses of up to 10 - 15 drops of a 1:5 dry or 1:2 fresh herb tincture may be taken orally immediately after the injury and again 6-8 hours later to prevent swelling and the myalgia that often follows the day after. (Moore) The homeopathic preparation is so safe and effective, that I find no need to use tincture of Arnica. Oral use of herbal Arnica should be avoided in patients with liver, kidney, or blood vessel disease. It is also contraindicated in the presence of gastro-intestinal inflammation and should not be applied topically to open wounds or abrasions. These contraindications do not apply to the homeopathic preparation, which can be ingested safely in any of these situations.

Topically, herbal preparations of either herbal or homeopathic Arnica help prevent and dispel the stagnation of blood and lymph fluids that often accumulate in the first 24 - 48 hours after an injury, although it is not as efficient at the job as the internally ingested homeopathic preparation. Infused herbal oils of Hypericum and Achillea are also useful topically and may be combined with the topical Arnica to enhance results. Neither of these latter herbs will cause problems in cases where the skin is broken, whereas topical applications of herbal Arnica is contraindicated in these cases. Yarrow (Achillea) is specifically indicated for open wounds where it promotes healing and acts as a disinfectant, anodyne when applied topically.

Arnica Case

One year while I was camping in the mountains with my little Peruvian mare, Rosa, I watched a fellow from a neighboring campsite get thrown high into the air when his young horse bucked hard and repeatedly. It was a long way to the ground and when the poor fellow landed, he hit hard! At first I was concerned about the possibility of serious internal injuries, as the man had the air knocked out of him and was initially unable to breathe. He recovered his breath quickly, much to everyone's relief, and was soon back on his feet and walking toward the offending horse, who eyed him with suspicion.

"You really hit hard!" I exclaimed in concern. "I have a homeopathic first aid remedy if you want to try some. It's totally safe and will help prevent the pain and swelling that you are likely to start feeling in a couple of hours."

True to his cowboy nature the man responded gruffly, "I'm fine. I don't need anything."

At that point I guessed his pride was hurting more than his body.

"OK," I replied, "but if you change your mind I will be back in camp again in about an hour and you are welcome to come by and get some."

"No, I'm fine," he insisted as he steadied his horse to climb back on.

He and his horse rode off without further incident but it is of interest to note that his response, insisting that he is fine, is typical of the initial state of shock and denial that occur when Arnica is just what we need.

A few hours later I noticed him limping around camp. He looked mighty sore to me, and I could only imagine how he actually felt.

"Are you sure you don't want some of that medicine?" I offered again. "I've got plenty of it in the truck."

"Yeah, sure, I'll take some."

Given the intensity of the fall, and the fact that it was now a few hours later instead of right after the injury, I decided to start with the highest potency I had on hand, a 50M. I gave him one dose then dispensed a vial of 200C to be taken every 4 hours for 24 hours then every 4 - 6 hours as needed after that. He took the medicine gratefully.

A few hours later, I was invited to join a group of campers around their fire. The cowboy and his buddies were also in attendance. He looked much better and expressed his gratitude.

"What is this stuff?" he asked. "It's amazing."

He actually ended up needing the 200C every 2 - 3 hours for that first 24 hours, which suggested to me that I should have given him a 1M to follow up with rather than the 200C.

On another occasion a young horse startled and threw his head, colliding with the rider's face. The rider's glasses were shoved upwards, resulting in a jagged laceration just above her left eye.

"You are going to need stitches for that laceration," I commented as I administered a 1M potency of Arnica.

Although she agreed, no one thought the wound critical enough to warrant shortening our ride, so she reported to the emergency room a few hours later, where she was dutifully sutured up. The attending physicians were surprised that she had not developed any discoloration or swelling at the site of injury, given how hard she had been hit. She later reported that the wound healed with surprising rapidity and she never did develop the black eye that would usually have accompanied such an injury.

Sprains and Strains

Acute sprains and strains of muscles and ligamentous tissues respond well to homeopathic medicine. As with most injuries, treatment should be initiated with Arnica, then once the first layer of trauma passes, the symptoms will often settle into another pattern. Occasionally, Arnica will be all that is needed, but many times another remedy picture will emerge.

Bryonia will be indicated when pain and discomfort are worse from even the slightest motion.

Rhus tox has been the most common second prescription to follow Arnica in my experience. This remedy does well when the patient's pain and/or stiffness and swelling are worse after rest and first movement, but better with continued motion as the affected area gets loosened up.

Ruta seems to work well when neither Bryonia nor Rhus tox are indicated, or symptoms are not well differentiated enough to point to either remedy. Ruta is an important medicine for ligaments and tendons.

Hydrotherapy should be initiated utilizing 20 minutes of ice or very cold applications in the initial 24 - 48 hours alternating with 20 minutes of no applications. It is important to remember that while cold applications initially vasoconstrict and reduce swelling and congestion, long term cold has the opposite effect, causing stagnation, so taking breaks from the cold pack every twenty minutes is very important if optimal healing is to be achieved.

Once the initial phase of inflammation and swelling is over, the use of alternating hot and cold applications will enhance circulation to the affected area. The treatment is started with a hot application which lasts 3 - 5 minutes, followed by a cold application for one minute. Alternating back and forth between hot and cold can be repeated several times and performed two or more times per day. The more difference there is between the hot and cold temperatures, the greater the beneficial effects of the treatment. The treatment should always be ended with the cold phase.

For sprains of ankles or wrists, two buckets can be used to do alternating hot and cold treatments. It is then very easy to alternate back and forth between the hot and cold.

Ruta Case

On another trip into the mountains, a friend's horse suddenly developed symptoms of acute tendinitis with heat and swelling in the lower aspect of one of his limbs. It was the first morning of the trip, so it was not due to overexertion. A veterinarian who happened to be on site confirmed the diagnosis. I dosed the horse with 10M Ruta every 4 hours for the first day then every 4 - 6 hours on the second, even getting up a few times that first night to check on him and repeat the dose. My friend did local poultices (I don't remember any more what she used) and the horse was already better the next day. A week later she was able to ride him 15 miles on the trails and the horse did fine.

Chronic tendinitis (in humans or animals) can be stubborn. Ruta 30C given 4 times a day usually clears up the problem, although Rhus tox may be indicated if symptoms are worse with first motion after a period of rest and better with continued motion. Anti-inflammatory foods and herbs such as turmeric, bromelain, adaptogens, and blueberries, among others, can be included to support the healing process. Treatment with therapeutic ultrasound can also be considered.

Calendula (Calendula officinalis) Asteraceae

A succus or juice of Calendula flowers has long been utilized as a vulnerary, where it acts as an excellent bacteriostatic disinfectant. Unlike commercial disinfectants, however, Calendula also promotes healing, soothes inflammation without suppressing, and minimizes the formation of scar tissue. Calendula succus was widely used as a surgical scrub in surgical procedures in Europe during WWII and during the Civil War here in the United States.

Calendula may be used topically for fresh wounds, burns, festering wounds, and on mucous membrane surfaces with catarrh and inflammation. The addition of Calendula to a formula including equal parts of Echinacea, Myrrh, and Hydrastis makes an excellent medicine for acute pharyngitis. Thirty to sixty drops of the herbal combination can be mixed with an ounce of water, gargled as a topical vulnerary for inflamed tissues of the pharynx, and then swallowed for further lymphatic and immune support.

Calendula has been used topically for glandular swellings and as one part of a whole protocol for treating basal cell carcinoma of the skin. As an herbal eyewash it combines well with goldenseal for the treatment of infectious conjunctivitis, although homeopathic Pulsatilla often clears up acute or chronic cases of conjunctivitis quite readily without the use of herbs.

Calendula may be used topically for bee stings, sprains, strains, and skin eruptions such as eczema and psoriasis where it soothes chronic inflammation and helps heal the skin without suppressing discharges.

Except in the most minor of wounds, Calendula should be taken internally as well as applied externally in which case the herb assists topical applications by preventing lymphatic stagnation and encouraging a positive immune response from within. Internal dosing also helps stave off the state of exhaustion that often follows the day after a significant injury. The herb has been used internally to treat low grade lingering wounds that are threatening to suppurate. It is particularly useful in these instances where lymphatic stagnation or swelling is part of the picture. In these latter cases, it should be combined with Echinacea and Baptisia.

Calendula contains some bitters, making it mildly active as a cholagogue. Over all, this plant acts as a gentle stimulant to the liver and digestive tract and can be trusted for the treatment of children or those less vital patients who might be bowled over by a stronger, more forceful liver herb. In chronic cases it is well indicated when a tendency to dampness exists, as with chronic mucous membrane catarrh, liver congestion, and chronic leucorrhea. It may be used both by mouth and as a douche in the treatment of vaginitis. Its antifungal actions make it useful for vaginitis where an overgrowth of Candida albicans is causing irritation. It is also efficacious when taken orally for the treatment of thrush, where it should be swished around in the mouth before being swallowed.

Culpepper writes that Calendula is a diaphoretic and will aid in bringing out the eruption in childhood exanthems such as measles. These diseases, once viewed as an avenue for the child's immature immune system to grow and develop, were benign in most cases, generally conferring lifelong immunity once the child had recovered. The eruption of the classic skin rash was accompanied by a disappearance of fever, myalgia, and fatigue. The rashes were considered a welcome sight, marking the end of the febrile stage and confirming the suspected diagnosis.

Calendula is said to strengthen and comfort the heart. The yellow or orange flowers close just prior to sunset and open again at sunrise. Like the sun whose path the flowers follow, Calendula brings light to those wet stagnant places, drying up the excess moisture and gently moving stagnation along. So too, Calendula brings herbal sunshine to the melancholic heart that is all the more saddened by cloudy days. The bright yellow and orange flowers are a cheery sight to see and if blossoms are regularly trimmed as they fade, the flowers will bloom all summer long.

"The Marigold that goes to bed with the sun,
And with him rises weeping." . . . . .William Shakespeare

Yarrow (Achillea millefolium) Asteraceae

This is a plant to restore the wounded healer and renew the wounded warrior. When the practitioner comes home heavily burdened by the stories and suffering of patients, yarrow is the herbal ally to cleanse, strengthen, and return the healer to balance. A comforting warm tea, drop doses of tincture (2 - 5 drops as desired), inhaling the scent of flowers and leaves, rubbing the herb on a part of the body, or placing it into a bath, can be combined with a bit of prayer to mend the spirit and rebuild boundaries and spiritual protection. A regular respectful relationship with the plant will enhance the protective power it offers to compassionate healers. In similar fashion yarrow can aid to restore the wounded warrior, those politically or socially active folks who take on the troubles of the world, as well as the emotionally or physically wounded soldier returning from the horrors of war.

Yarrow flower essence is specific for those sensitive folks who are overly vulnerable to environmental toxins, whether of physical, mental, emotional, or spiritual origin.

As a first aid herb, yarrow is invaluable for staunching the wounds of the "weekend warrior" who ends up flying off his bike or snowboard, or for the inveterate equine addict who gets herself blasted by tree branches hanging along the forest path as her mighty steed gallops along. Matthew Wood differentiates yarrow from arnica, when he suggests that while both herbs are indicated for bruising and soft tissue injuries, arnica is contraindicated whenever skin or mucous membranes are broken. Yarrow, on the other hand, is just the plant for the more "violent" cuts and breaks in the skin. (Remember homeopathic Arnica taken internally is completely safe in any of these circumstances.)

Flowering tops may be dried and ground into a powder to keep handy in the first aid kit. When needed, the powdered herb can be placed directly onto the wound, where it acts as a styptic, anti-inflammatory, disinfectant, and local decongestant. I have watched this herb miraculously take down rapidly mounting swelling, bleeding, and bruising when the poultice was applied immediately after the injury. It will sometimes dissipate pain just as instantaneously. Amazing little plant, I wish I were half the healer these little green folks are!

YARROW CASE

Several years ago, I woke with inflammation and joint pain that were uncharacteristic for me. As I journeyed in to my symptoms, I found myself thinking of a dear friend I knew who was struggling with significant arthritis. For some reason, my body was picking something up to help her. Fortunately, I happened to have the day off, and although I went about my day as usual, I took extra time to pray for her, for whatever she needed, and did a small ceremony to ground whatever healing I could for her, and for anyone else who shared her problem.

Throughout the day, I kept craving a cup of yarrow tea, but as I was busy with farm chores and training a young horse, I never quite got to it. At 3 o'clock in the afternoon, I settled on the couch to read Matthew Woods' then new book "The Book of Herbal Wisdom," and was thrilled to see that the first chapter was a discussion of Achillea (yarrow). The craving for a cup of yarrow tea grew stronger as I commenced reading. When I came to his description of the use of a yarrow poultice for the topical first aid treatment of wounds, I thought, "Oh, I have to remember to try that sometime!"

Little did I know how soon my opportunity would arrive!

The horses were loose on the lawn that day and at 4 o'clock, my hungry young colt, Waku, appeared at the window demanding his dinner. I reluctantly set the book down and headed out to feed.

Now normally, I would lock each horse into their individual stalls before fetching their hay, which was an especially wise practice with this feisty colt, but on that particular day, impatient to get back to my book, I just grabbed a couple flakes of hay from the barn while Waku was still loose and walked it to the stall with him at my side.

Well, what can I say? No one is wise all the time! The hungry little colt grabbed for some hay, missed, and bit the back of my hand. I rewarded him by dumping the hay into the stall, then after feeding the mares, headed into the house in search of the yarrow.

I was so eager to try the poultice that I didn't even put pressure on the wound. It was only a superficial flesh wound, but it was bleeding pretty profusely. I tossed my dried yarrow flowers into the blender, ground them into a powder then dumped the whole lot onto my hand.

The results were astonishing. Not only did the fairly profuse bleeding stop instantly, but all the swelling and bruising that were beginning to show under the skin around the laceration, visibly faded away. Then, as suddenly as it had appeared, the joint pain I had been struggling with all day vanished. Yarrow, the herb for the wounded healer, cleared the symptoms from my body that were not mine to continue carrying.

Burns

Many plants have been used for the topical treatment of burns, including St. John's Wort (Hypericum perforatum) and Calendula, but my unwavering favorite in this instance is the inner gel of the aloe vera plant. Aloe vera juice contains a polysaccharide, glucomannin, which is particularly active as a vulnerary.

The essential oil of Lavender has also been used successfully in treating burns. Lavender is unusually safe as essential oils go, but because this oil is safe does not mean another essential oil will do as well. Care should be taken when using essential oils as many will irritate and burn healthy skin. Lavender is the only essential oil that I am aware of that is safe in the treatment of burns.

Homeopathic Cantharis is often helpful for burns. Frequent dosing of a 6, 12, or 30C potency as needed for pain can be miraculous at eradicating the discomfort of a burn. In cases where it does relieve pain, it will also facilitate more rapid healing, especially if used in conjunction with the herbs. More severe burns should be treated with higher potencies.

Cantharis 6, 12 or 30C will also help facilitate healing and alleviate pain after cauterization of sun damaged skin lesions by the dermatologist.

Recently, after spilling a cup of hot soup on my lap, I learned that the topical use of peppermint tooth paste placed immediately on a burn will have an immediate cooling effect, reducing pain as it pulls heat from the affected area. Special thanks to my friend and colleague, Nathalie Paravacini N.D., for this tip that stems from her childhood in Venezuela.

It is best NOT to use infused oils for topical application in the early stages of a burn, as the oils may lock in heat and interfere with normal cooling mechanisms.

Infected Wounds

Antibiotics are rarely necessary in treating infected wounds if the practitioner is familiar with a few simple homeopathic remedies.

While there are a number of remedies to consider in these cases, those listed below will serve most of the time.

In the absence of constitutional symptoms such as fever, chills, red streaks, or significant lymphadenopathy, Hepar Sulph will usually be of service in clearing up infection. The site will be red and tender to the touch and there may be some purulent discharge. If the development of infection has been slow or is of a more chronic nature, or Hepar sulph does not seem to be doing the trick, Silicea should be considered.

If chilling, weakness, alternating sensations of heat and chill, and pale facial color, accompany infection, consider Pyrogenium. Although one would expect a fever in such cases, often there is no rise in temperature when this remedy is indicated and in fact there may even be a subnormal temperature. Boericke describes this phenomenon as "adynamic fever" in his materia medica of homeopathic remedies. The presence of fever does not contraindicate the use of this remedy however, even if the fever runs high.

Homeopathic Belladonna should be given for the first stage of inflammation or cellulitis, where there is no discharge but the tissues are unusually bright red. One of the other above mentioned remedies may be needed 24 - 48 hours after Belladonna has stopped working if Belladonna alone does not cure the case.

Homeopathic Baptisia should also be considered. Although I have no personal experience using this particular remedy for the treatment of infected wounds, it is in the literature and I have had great success in using it herbally for infected tissues, where it combines exceedingly well with Echinacea.

Other remedies to consider include Anthrocynum and Myristica, although these remedies have not been as common in my practice.

Acute abscesses will generally respond well to Hepar sulph, although Calc sulph may be the appropriate remedy on some occasions. Silica should be given whenever abscess tends towards chronicity or if there is not the desired response to other remedies. Tooth abscesses often respond to Hepar Sulph or Mercurius.

Spider bites can be treated with a clay poultice wetted down with a strong decoction or tincture of Echinacea. This simple treatment will work better if the topical application is accompanied by internal administration of Echinacea tincture at doses of 60 drops every two hours for a couple days then every four hours until symptoms subside.

As with any acute condition, a 30C of the indicated remedy can be given every 2 - 4 hours for 24 hours or a 200C every 4 - 8 hours tapering as symptoms improve. Frequency of dosing is dependent on severity of symptoms. Amelioration should be seen in 24 hours in acute cases if the correct remedy has been administered. If the abscess is more chronic, calling for a remedy like Silica, it might be necessary to give it more time. Silica abscesses will present with more low grade symptoms, so waiting a few extra days is not as critical as with an acutely painful abscess. It may be necessary to continue Silica for 3 to 7 days or even longer before deciding to move on to another remedy. Silica may be dosed at a 30C 2 - 4 times daily or a 200C 1 - 2 times per day for a few days, as the abscess calling for Silica is often more low grade and chronic. Sometimes an even lower potency such as 6C or 12C may be given 2 -4 times daily for a longer period.

The use of herbal preparations of Echinacea and Baptisia tinctoria (wild indigo) will enhance the healing process initiated by homeopathic prescribing through improving immune response, decreasing lymphatic stagnation, and addressing underlying issues of toxicity. Echinacea, well known as an immune stimulant is also a powerful blood cleanser. It is especially well indicated for staph, strep and suppurating wounds.

The addition of Baptisia tinctoria potentizes the effects of Echinacea in infection and sepsis. The Eclectic physician Felter describes the specific indications for Baptisia well when he writes that the herb should be considered for "Fetid discharges … tendency to ulceration and decay … sepsis … fullness of tissues ... ulcers of an indolent character, with bluish or purplish edges."

Baptisia is a strong botanical and should be dosed judiciously. An average adult dose of a 1:1 fresh herb tincture may be dosed at 10 drops 4 times per day. Like most plants, the first signs of toxicity are nausea and vomiting. Should a person continue to consume the herb despite these warning symptoms, tachycardia and ultimately respiratory arrest may ensue. The herb is entirely safe when dispensed in proper doses

Drawing poultices of grated raw potato, slippery elm powder, or Epsom salts will aid in facilitating the removal of purulent matter from the wound, but the most powerful poultice in my experience is made from the simple leaves of fresh plantain, whose drawing power exceeds that of any other substances I have had occasion to try for such purposes.

It is important to avoid the use of comfrey topically on any wound that is likely to be infected. Comfrey's ability to heal is so rapid that it has been known to seal infection in.

Plantain (Plantago lanceolata, Plantago major) Plantaginaceae

Plantain is common in lawns, waysides, and pastures. Native to Europe, it became known in North America as white man's footprint, popping up wherever white newcomers appeared.

Plantain has gained status as a superlative agent for drawing toxins, pus, or foreign objects from wounds, a reputation that is well deserved. Fresh leaves should be chewed in the mouth to break down the cell walls of the plant and release the healing constituents. Once macerated the plant is then placed on an insect bite or bee sting to bring relief and pull venom from the site. Historically it has been used topically for curing snake bite. The leaf is cooling, astringent, and mildly styptic as well as drawing.

Plantain has more potential for use as medicine than most of us give it credit for. In the Scottish Highlands it was (and may still be) known as the "Plant of Healing," while the Saxons listed it among their nine sacred herbs. (Grieve) It is not infrequently found in old formulas. The leaves are mucilaginous as well as astringent, making them useful for respiratory and urinary tract conditions. It acts as a cooling anti-inflammatory demulcent when an infusion is applied to the eyes and it has anti-bacterial properties, particularly with regard to Staph aureus. It may be taken for conditions affecting the digestive tract, or any mucous membranes where it acts as an astringent, demulcent, and anti-inflammatory.

Long attracted to the simple plantain, I was struck when an article appeared in The Letter for Doctors[76] in which the writer described a case of a man with AIDS who began to take one leaf of plantago lanceolata, pour a cup of boiling water over it and drink it each night at bedtime. His long term lymphadenopathy, tendency to infection, and general fatigue cleared up. He continued it for some time, finally backing off some months later only to have his former symptoms return. His symptoms again resolved upon restarting the tea.

The writer, who did not have AIDS and was not HIV positive, tried it on herself for some vague immune problems with similar results. Although as the writer herself pointed out, these are only two incidents, they do suggest that we may not be recognizing all the potential healing contained within this common little invader.

Since reading this article I have, on several occasions, dosed myself with a simple tea of fresh leaves of Plantago lanceolata for symptoms of myalgia, low energy, and mild respiratory symptoms consistent with an acute viral syndrome such as an impending cold or flu. I have found the herb to be a reliable ally in alleviating my complaints quite quickly when taken at the first sign of symptoms. I have no idea if tincture or capsules of dried herb would be as effective, but the tea definitely seems to have some influence.

Case: Acute abscess

I walked out to the paddock to collect my mare April Moon for a ride one morning only to find her unwilling to put even the slightest amount of weight on her right front foot. Suspecting a hoof abscess, I gave her a dose of Hepar Sulph 200C and haltered up my colt for a lesson in the round pen, forgoing my ride in the woods on April. An hour later, as I finished up with the colt, April whinnied at me demanding to get out on the trail. A little surprised, I looked up to see her walking totally normally. Clearly the Hepar sulph was the right remedy for the problem! Despite the dramatic improvement and her continued insistence that we get out on the trail, I decided we would still take the day off from riding. The abscess never returned.

Another horse who was well into her twenties and had been immunized religiously every year by her well meaning owner, presented with a chronic low grade hoof abscess that never came to a head and never cleared up. The mare had been off and on lame for 3 or 4 years by the time I met her. An initial dose of the obvious homeopathic remedy, Silica, did nothing. After thinking about the case a bit more I decided to give her homeopathic Thuja, a remedy that is specific for over vaccination. The mare was stand offish and aloof, suspicious of others, and did not even connect to the other horses normally, all confirmatory signs for a homeopathic prescription of Thuja. A dose of 200C was given and although the abscess remained unchanged a subtle shift in her energy suggested the remedy had acted.

The homeopathic Silica was then repeated a month later and cured the abscess, although several doses were needed before the case was complete.

Here was a case where immune suppression from overvaccination prevented the Silica from acting until the remedy for the etiology of immune suppression was given.

Case: Cat Bite

Some years ago a cat I was transporting to the veterinarian for euthanasia bit me when my hand inadvertently slipped into his wound as the car lurched over a bump in the road. The cat had a huge open gash on his side that was simply not healing due to immune suppression from other causes. Unfortunately, despite all my caution, my hand slipped in such a way that it fell right into the very wound I was trying so hard to protect. The cat, normally very tolerant and loving, reacted in pain and sunk his incisor full length into my hand, then froze for what seemed like an eternity.

Cat's mouths are well known to be crawling with particularly pathogenic bacteria, and the wound from such a bite is a closed puncture wound, making it even worse. Once the cat was taken care of, the friend I was with drove me to my office, where I was able to administer a tetanus vaccine for myself and gather a few herbs together, Echinacea in the form of Optibiotics (available from Eclectic Institute in Sandy, Oregon), Baptisia, and some extra Vitamin C, all of which I started immediately.

By eight o'clock that evening I was pretty ill. My hand was hot, red, and swollen and I felt sick with fever and chills. The infection felt like it was progressing quickly and I worried that I might end up in the hospital on IV antibiotics. Because the wound was septic, accompanied by constitutional symptoms of fever and chills, I chose homeopathic Pyrogen. One dose of a 10M potency brought relief within 5 - 10 minutes. Pain, swelling, and redness began to subside as did symptoms of fever and chilling. I continued the remedy in that potency as needed every 4 - 8 hours with complete resolution of symptoms.

Fractures

The soft tissue injury that always accompanies fractures should be treated with homeopathic Arnica as soon as possible after the incident. A 200C or a 1M should be taken every 4 hours for 24 hours while the patient is awake, followed by every 6 - 8 hours for 24 hours, then only as needed for soft tissue pain and swelling.

The Arnica should be alternated with Eupatorium perfoliatum 200C which is taken every 4 hours or more often as needed for bone pain. This remedy is so effective at relieving fracture pain that the need for pharmaceutical medications is often circumvented altogether. The plant Eupatorium perfoliatum, from which the remedy is prepared, is specifically indicated for flu symptoms where there is aching deep to the bone.

On occasion there may be enough pain from strained tendons or ligaments that homeopathic Ruta will need to be alternated with the Eupatorium, although generally pain from connective tissue injury comes later, after Arnica and Eupatorium perfoliatum have finished their work.

Although I have no experience with it, some homeopaths use Symphytum for bone pain. Dosing for acute fracture pain should be the same as with Eupatorium. Herbally Symphytum officinalis, more commonly known as comfrey, can be very effective as a topical agent in encouraging bone healing. Chopped root is laid on the skin over the site of the fracture, or a fresh leaf can be lightly steamed and laid over the site.

Although comfrey has traditionally been used internally over long periods of time for a multitude of problems, it does contain pyrrolizidine alkaloids, which can cause severe veno-occlusive liver disease in some individuals. Our modern livers, overtaxed with the heavy load of toxins in the environment, are not as able to process these alkaloids as our ancestors once could. Sadly, the internal use of pyrrolizidine alkaloid containing plants is no longer recommended. If the patient has sustained a rib fracture, homeopathic Bryonia, prepared from the plant of the same name, will serve better.

Bone Broth Recipe

1) Place marrow rich bones from any meat into a pot, cover with water, and add a teaspoon or so of vinegar.
2) Bring the whole thing to a boil, skim then allow simmering for 8 to 24 hours. Longer immersion and simmering extracts more minerals from bone and marrow.
3) Bone broth may be prepared either in a crock pot or on the stove and will be highly nourishing for healing fractured bones or in rebuilding bones in osteoporosis.

Herbs high in minerals can be made into a strong tea and sipped throughout the day. A quart jar should be filled 1/3 full of a combination of nettle leaves, (Urtica dioica), horsetail herb (Equisetum arvense), dandelion leaves (Taraxacum officinalis), and gotu kola (Centella asiatica). All these herbs are rich in minerals, while gotu kola may also aid in preventing excessive scar tissue from developing. The jar is then filled with water that has been brought to a boil and the infusion is left to sit overnight. Alternatively, hot bone broth can be poured over the herbs and left to sit for 20 - 45 minutes. The herbs are then strained off and the bone broth tea may be drunk as a soup 2 - 4 times per day or the simple tea can be drunk throughout the day.

Alternatively a vinegar preparation may be made by placing the herbal mix into a jar and covering with apple cider vinegar that has been brought to a boil. The vinegar extracts the minerals from the herbs, something that does not happen in an alcoholic extract. This mix should be allowed to sit in a dark place for six weeks before being strained for use, making it more practical for the treatment of osteoporosis than an acute fracture. The acidic content of the vinegar extract also aids in assimilation of minerals in the body. Assimilation of both protein and minerals will be hindered in the patient with hypochlorhydria or low stomach acid.

Dried nettles leaves go unnoticed in scrambled eggs, stir-fries, salads, and soups and can be used in this way in addition to the tea. Nettles leaves also alkalinize the blood, enabling the body to neutralize and eliminate toxins more readily, always a help in enhancing the healing process.

Other herbs high in minerals include seaweeds and raspberry leaves. The silica content of horsetail and nettles is particularly valuable in building good bone.

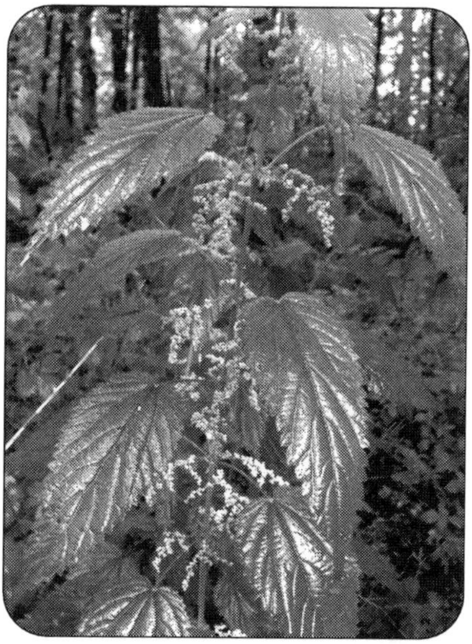

Nettles

Photo courtesy of Mark Greg Iwanicki

It is vital that the diet be adequate in good quality protein as protein is essential for building the matrix within bone tissue that the minerals are set upon. Adequate protein is also important for wound healing and prevention of infection.

Case: Fracture

A long time patient reported to clinic for help with fracture pain after being seen in the emergency room where the fracture of the 5th metacarpal of the right hand had been set. The patient had been given a prescription of codeine for the pain but was reluctant to use it as she tended to be highly sensitive to drugs and was very fearful of taking the codeine, despite intense pain at the site of injury.

"I know you have something else," she said tearfully as she told her story. "I'm just so afraid to take these drugs!"

After reassuring her, I prescribed Arnica 200C to be taken as needed for soft tissue pain which was to be alternated with Eupatorium perfoliatum 200C for bone pain.

A day or two later the young woman called the office, jubilant with the success of the homeopathic treatment.

"These remedies are working great!" she exclaimed over the phone. "I haven't felt the need for that codeine at all!"

Tetanus Toxoid

Although I am not a big proponent of vaccines, Clostridium tetani, the bacteria that causes tetanus, is widespread in our soils and the disease can be serious, very painful, and life threatening. If the patient, adult or child, has not been fully immunized at the time of an injury, it is too late to immunize at that point and the only alternative that will be offered is gamma globulin, a blood product far more fraught with risk than the simple series of vaccines for tetanus. Although tetanus vaccines are not without risk, they generally have a good safety record, and are a better bet than either the gamma globulin or the disease.

Chapter 11

Pelvic Decongestant Herbs for Men and Women

THIS GROUP OF HERBS ENCOURAGES THE FLOW OF ENERGY, blood, and lymph through the pelvis, enhancing the delivery of nutrients and removal of toxic waste products from the area. These herbs are important in treating any condition in the pelvis, including ovarian symptoms, menstrual cramps, uterine fibroids, endometriosis, dysfunctional uterine bleeding, amenorrhea, recurrent or chronic urinary symptoms, and in men, prostate symptoms, epididymitis, orchitis, urethral irritation, and erectile dysfunction.

A well indicated pelvic decongestant herb can be given as a simple or in formulas of 3 - 4 well indicated complimentary herbs. Tinctures of simples or formulated herbs can then be dosed at 30 to 60 drops 3 to 4 times per day.

Kegels, pelvic floor exercises, yoga, horseback riding, visceral manipulation, Maya abdominal massage and belly dancing can also be helpful in keeping life generating energy flowing through the pelvis.

Achillea millefolium (Yarrow) Asterceae

Flowers and leaves of wild yarrow are valuable as an astringent for hemorrhagic menses. The plant's styptic actions may also be useful in bleeding from the urinary or gastro-intestinal tracts. Yarrow is anti-inflammatory and may serve well in ovarian inflammation, chronic urinary tract infections, and interstitial cystitis. It has also been used in formulas for fibroid tumors of the uterus, a condition often accompanied by overly heavy bleeding. Where menses are delayed or sluggish in onset, yarrow may be used as an emmenogogue to encourage the flow.

As discussed earlier, yarrow is especially indicated for those sensitive folks who are highly affected by the external environment. In this regard it is specific for the compassionate wounded healer who comes home after a long day of open hearted listening, carrying too many of the stories and emotional, or even physical, pains of their patients.

Yarrow also lends strength and protection to the wounded warrior, where it helps stem the emotional hemorrhage of the social activist, spiritual warrior, or soldier who feels worn down and battered from "fighting the good fight." Yarrow is the herb to make the healer/warrior whole again.

Bitter constituents in yarrow stimulate digestion and liver function. As a hot tea, it is often recommended at the first sign of cold or flu for its diaphoretic action. In these cases, it has most often been combined with elder flower. A cold infusion is said to work as a diuretic.

Actea racemosa/Cimicifuga (Black Cohosh) Ranunculaceae

Black cohosh, well known for its actions in the female reproductive tract, is specifically indicated for deep dark depression, especially when accompanied by a history of sexual or physical abuse, psychic attack or trauma, or a history of substance abuse either in the patient or in a close family member. Depression can be constant or come in sudden waves that envelop the patient in a dark cloud of gloom and despair. There may or may not be an associated wild feeling in the mind, with difficulty in focusing, irritability, and loquacity.

Actea is an invaluable ally for the woman whose descent into the underworld of sexual abuse, incest, and domestic violence, mirrors the journey of the Greek goddess Persephone. As a maiden, this goddess was abducted and taken into the underworld by the dark god Hades, after her father sold her out in exchange for the gold that was buried in Hades' underworld depths.

Like the woman whose incestuous father betrays his innocent daughter to his own lascivious dark side because he cannot, or will not, face the Hades within himself, Zeus sacrifices Persephone to feed his greed for gold.

Persephone is eventually released when the intercession of two other goddesses creates enough pressure on Zeus that he finally orders her to be freed from the clutches of the underworld. On the way out, however, Persephone, who has hitherto partaken of neither food nor drink during her stay in the underworld, impulsively eats one pomegranate seed. As a result, she is required to return to the underworld for part of each year, but this time when she descends, she returns as Queen. No longer a victim, Persephone now descends to serve as a guide and source of solace for other souls who are forced to make the descent. Her time in the underworld is marked on the earth by the season of winter while summer reflects her stay above ground and autumn and spring indicate her descent and reemergence from the underworld.

The pomegranate fruit, bursting with seeds that drip a burgundy red flavonoid-rich juice is often compared to the ovary, full of seeds that promise new life and not coincidentally, pomegranates are associated with fertility. Persephone's decision to eat the seeds of the pomegranate reflects her choice to accept the cycles of life, which include dark challenges as well as light.

Like the Goddess Herself, Actea can be an incredible ally to help clear away murky clouds of despair and delusion, mobilizing the underworld traveler as it mobilizes energy through the pelvis. In cases where depression is more pressing, Actea can be given as a simple with instructions to take a few drops by mouth as needed for feelings of despair, agitation, and hopelessness. It also combines well with a small amount of kava, which helps to lift the patient up to "Eagle Vision," adding mental clarity and a larger, more enlightened perspective on the process. Flower essences can be added, such as mustard for depression, agrimony for a sense of torment, or sweet chestnut for anguish.

A few drops of the formula can be taken as often as needed. Although toxicity is highly unlikely at these low doses, the patient should be instructed to back off dosing if a dull frontal headache occurs. In the past, I prescribed doses of 30 drops as needed of either Actea alone or the formula. Even at these doses, the dull headache was rare, making it highly unlikely at low drop doses. In more recent years, I have discovered that the low drop doses work equally well for most patients struggling with depression and agitation.

As a pelvic herb, Actea can be used all month long for the treatment of menstrual cramps, where it acts to tone the uterine muscle, relieve pelvic congestion, and act as an anti-spasmodic and anti-inflammatory. It is especially well suited when menstrual pain radiates to cause an achy sensation in the low back or down the legs. Despite its general reputation as an anti-spasmodic, it is also used to strengthen contractions in labor.

The plant is best indicated as an emmenogogue for scanty or late menses or for amenorrhea, although heavy menses does not necessarily contraindicate its use. It can be very helpful for the prevention and treatment of menstrual migraines in certain cases. Here it should be compared with feverfew, lavender, and western coltsfoot.

Actea is often very effective for menopausal symptoms. Hot flashes, insomnia, depression, and mood swings can all he helped by the addition of this herb. Black coshosh may be used intravaginally in combination with Vitamin E for atrophic changes in the vagina and has been shown in multiple studies to be protective in the prevention of osteoporosis.[77,78]

Current research suggests that constituents of Actea compete for binding at estrogen receptor sites on the cells, thereby normalizing estrogen metabolism and making it useful for hyperestrogenic conditions such as endometriosis as well as for the treatment of menopausal complaints.

Actea is not just an herb for women. Pelvic congestion in men with prostatitis or epididymitis may also be helped by this plant, especially if there is an achy pain in prostate or testicles or the patient presents with the mental symptoms calling for its use.

Skeletal muscle spasm responds well to the addition of Actea where again the herb acts to relieve spasm and soothe inflammation. Rheumatic symptoms, including joint pain, arthritis, and fibromyalgia, are covered by Actea's anti-inflammatory properties.

The achiness that is experienced by the patient needing Actea is reflected in its use as a remedy for the early stages of influenza, where it also acts as an expectorant. It has been used in the treatment of asthma and asthmatic bronchitis to relax the bronchioles, relieve inflammation and act as a bronchodilatior.

Actea may also be used in the treatment of hypertension, where it acts to relax smooth muscles in vessel walls and encourage peripheral vasodilation. It is anti-spasmodic, anti-inflammatory, tonic to the reproductive tract and nervous system, and decongestant. In addition, Actea has actions as a diaphoretic, diuretic, and mild digestive aid. It is contraindicated in the first trimester of pregnancy largely due to a possible abortifacient effect.

Roots are used for medicine and constituents include isoflavones, salicylic acid, triterpene glycosides, ferulic acid, isoferulic acid.

Signs of overdose of Actea include a dull frontal headache, usually the first symptom, which can proceed to a pounding headache if the herb is continued. I often administer Actea as a simple for the treatment of menopausal hot flashes, instructing the woman to dose the herb as needed to control flushes of heat, starting at a dose of 15 drops 3 times per day and moving up, warning them to back off if that dull frontal headache shows itself.

Further symptoms of toxicity that can appear in serious overdose include bradycardia, hypotension, nausea and vomiting, flushed face, a sensation of lightheadedness, and dilated pupils.

Please use farmed Actea whenever practical, as this plant is very popular and therefore may be in some danger of being overharvested.

Formula for Depression

The following formula is a template and should be adjusted as needed for each individual. The main herbs are the Actea/Cimicifuga and Piper.

The carnivorous herbs (Drosera, Dionaea muscipula, Sarracenia) "eat" negativity. As the carnivorous herbs are fragile and not commonly found in nature, please use tiny doses to synergize the formula. Larger doses are not necessary for the spiritual/emotional healing that is called for in these cases. The formula will still be effective if carnivorous herbs are unavailable.

The first 3 herbs provide the basic template. Other herbs listed below can be included as indicated.

Actea/Cimicifuga
Piper methysticum
Drosera, Sarracenia, or Dionaea muscipula, few drops per ounce
Crataegus for grief, closed heart, betrayal
Oplopanax for protection and empowerment
Hypericum to support anti-depressant activity

Flower Essences 2 drops of each per ounce:

Mustard for depression from unknown causes
Gentian for depression from self doubt
Agrimony for sense of torment
Sweet Chestnut for feelings of anguish

Dosage is 2 - 4 drops several times per day and as needed for depression. It works best if taken often throughout the day.

Angelica sinensis (Dong Quai/Chinese Angelica) *Umbelliferae*

Angelica is full of nutrients including calcium, magnesium, biotin, and vitamins B-12, C, E and A. It is a warming blood mover that promotes circulation to the pelvis, and nourishes and purifies the blood. As a uterine tonic, anti-inflammatory, and anti-spasmodic it may be taken all month to prevent menstrual cramps. As an alterative it may be helpful in regulating cycles. The herb is well known for its use as a nourishing tonic during the menopausal transition.

Nourishing blood building actions make Angelica especially well suited for women who feel weak and anemic during menses, even though the flow may be scanty. This herb is really not the best choice when menstrual flow tends to be heavy and is contraindicated in menorrhagia. Many herbalists recommend stopping the herb during menses, and restarting it once the flow has ceased.

Angelica is protective to the liver, a valuable function in these toxic times. It is indicated for constipation with hard dry stools where there is also pelvic stagnation. It should be considered for that peculiar type of constipation that accompanies older age, with dry hard stools and not much action. Dryness is a symptom that calls for this plant, hence its popularity for menopause.

Blood moving actions are not limited to the pelvis. Angelica increases blood flow through the coronary arteries, improving heart muscle contractility and decreasing arrhythmias. It should be considered for the treatment of angina, where it may be taken regularly to prevent episodes of chest pain. Dilation of peripheral vessels results in a lower blood pressure when hypertension is an issue and the presence of beta-sitosterol is thought to be a contributing factor to the mild cholesterol lowering effect seen with this plant.

Anti-spasmodic and anti-inflammatory qualities may aid in relaxing the smooth muscles of the bronchioles in cases of asthma.

Constituents include coumarins, phytosterols, ferulic acid, succinic acid, and sesquiterpenes. It is the roots of the plant that are used in medicine.

Angelica sinensis may cause or aggravate gastro-esophogeal reflux in some individuals. It may be contraindicated in patients on blood thinning pharmaceuticals as it contains coumarins. Furocoumarins can also create photosensitivity in some individuals.

Alchemilla vulgaris (Lady's Mantle) Rosaceae

Native to Europe, the soft, circular, fanned leaves and protective flavonoids of the lovely Alchemilla offer a magical mantle of shelter to women when an insensitive partner or abusive situation renders her more vulnerable to be hurt, emotionally as well as physically. It helps strengthen and protect the heart in these cases, physically and energetically. The morning dew that collects on the leaves in droplets is reputed to have magical healing properties, hence the name, Alchemilla.

Alchemilla acts as a gentle, restorative guardian after trauma. Here she helps to strengthen and protect the heart while offering emotional and spiritual protection. Following a severe accident, injury, or loss, normal boundaries are often shattered and inappropriate comments, innocently and unconsciously made by well meaning folks, can cut to the quick where they would normally pass unnoticed. Alchemilla offers shelter during sensitive moments, soothing shattered nerves in the process.

In the pelvis Alchemilla should be considered after the trauma of miscarriage, abortion, surgery, ruptured ovarian cyst, or pelvic inflammatory disease as well as following sexual transgressions or threats.

Lady's mantle is an excellent muscle tonic for uterus, heart, and abdominal muscles. Here it is more specifically indicated for conditions of laxity than hypertonicity. The plant has been used post partum to restore tone to uterine and abdominal muscles and to breasts after months of nursing. For the latter, it may be applied externally as a poultice as well as taken internally. It is also used all month long to tone the uterine muscle in treating menstrual cramps.

Nervine properties make the plant useful for premenstrual tension. Tannins lend astringency where heavy uterine bleeding is a problem or whenever excessively wet vaginal discharges occur due to laxity of tissues. Like its leaves that repel the water of rain and dew, Alchemilla tightens mucous membranes and repels excess fluid. Alchemilla can also be used to help regulate menstrual cycles.

Current literature suggests lady's mantle may possess significant anti-oxidant activity due at least in part to the presence of flavonoids.[79] Other constituents include tannins, salicylic acid, and a small amount of bitters.

Capsella bursa-pastoris (Shepherd's Purse) Brassicaceae

Shepherd's purse is used for uterine hemorrhage, and may be effective in staunching acute bleeding or taken all month to tonify uterine tissue and prevent excessive menstrual bleeding. It also acts as a gentle stimulant to the urinary tract. Aerial parts with the fruiting "little purses" must be used or tinctured fresh for the plant to be effective.

When used for menorrhagia (excessively heavy menstrual bleeding), it is best to dose all month in a low dose, increasing frequency and amounts as needed.

Caulophyllum thalictroides (Blue Cohosh) Berberidaceae

Caulophyllum helps ease ovarian symptoms and chronic inflammation. It is specific after acute PID (pelvic inflammatory disease) or ovarian congestion with mid-cycle achiness.

Although listed in many references as an anti-spasmodic, the plant is actually tonic to uterine muscle where it is used to stimulate contractions in labor or ease spasm in hypertonic uterine muscles. Menstrual cramps accompanied by a sensation of achy heaviness and dragging in the pelvis should bring blue cohosh to mind. Like all tonic herbs, the plant is best taken all month to prevent cramps.

Caulophyllum is indicated when there is profuse bleeding at menstruation or when menses appear too early. Alternatively it has been used as an emmenogogue for amenorrhea and delayed or suppressed menses.

The roots of Caulophyllum are used for medicine. The berries are poisonous and should not be used. Root constituents include alkaloids and saponins.

Caulophyllum is contraindicated in the early stages of pregnancy as it may induce miscarriage due to uterine stimulant actions. This having been said, it actually takes high, toxic doses of the herb to deliberately induce abortion in early stages of pregnancy. Please do not try this without supervision from an experienced practitioner.

Ceanothus spp. (Red Root, Wild Lilac) Rhamnaceae

Although Ceanothus americanus (New Jersey Tea) is the species most commonly cited in the books, there are at least 30-35 species of Ceanothus in North America, most of which can be used in medicine.

Ceanothus is abundant in nature and varies in presentation from a small bushy herb to a fairly large shrub. A nitrogen-fixing plant, Ceanothus often materializes to heal the land in overly disturbed areas. In Southern Oregon, plants can grow to be 4 - 6 feet in height and bushes may be found growing close to one another, intertwining to create an impassable thicket that protects the land from further intrusion. Leaves are small and flowers can be lusciously aromatic or not, appearing in blue, lavender, or white. The red-colored root bark is used most commonly, although leaves are also employed.

Other common names for species include buckbrush, wild lilac, deerbrush, and red root.

Although I have generally found a dose of 15 drops of tincture (1:4 dried herb) three items daily to be better than higher doses, it can be taken as high as 40 - 60 drops 3 - 4 times per day. If taken as a tea, 1-2 cups per day using 1 teaspoon of herb per cup of water can be taken. Moore recommends the cold infusion, which is prepared by allowing the herb to sit in cold water rather than the usual boiled water used to make teas.

Toxicity of Ceanothus is low. Constituents include flavonoids, triterpenes, methyl salicylate, resins, tannins, oils, a number of acids, and several alkaloids.

Lymph, liver, spleen, pelvic organs, respiratory tract, blood vessels, and circulation are all helped by Ceanothus when the symptom picture of congestion predominates. Ceanothus can be especially helpful in cases where stagnation of blood and lymph in the pelvis, combined with some degree of liver sluggishness, manifests in symptoms of menorrhagia (hemorrhagic menses), ovarian cysts, or fibroid tumors of the uterus. The astringent properties of tannins present in Ceanothus help staunch profuse bleeding while flavonoids compliment the styptic action by addressing capillary fragility.

Because Ceanothus acts as a tonic, it is best dosed all month long to treat the underlying tendency to menorrhagia. Mobilization of stagnant fluids in the pelvis encourages resolution of cysts by enhancing the flow of toxins out of reproductive tissues while increasing the supply of nutrient rich blood to the pelvis. In men, Ceanothus may prove useful in treating testicular hydroceles. (Moore)

Premenstrual breast tenderness is greatly helped by 15 drops of a tincture of Ceanothus given all month long. Breast tissue is highly lymphatic, thus the herb's action as a lymph mover, combined with its ability to support optimal liver function, makes it remarkably effective in resolving lymphatic congestion in breast tissues.

Mononucleosis, caused by an acute infection with Epstein Barr Virus, often presents with elevated liver enzymes and hepato-splenomegaly, as well as swollen lymph glands. Chronic infection with Epstein Barr Virus (EBV) can manifest as Chronic Fatigue Immunodeficiency Syndrome (CFIDS). Ceanothus is a specific for EBV, acute or chronic, where it improves immune function and decreases congestion in the spleen, liver and lymphatic systems in both chronic and acute infections.

Stimulation of digestive function also occurs with Ceanothus, not so much as a direct action on the digestive tract, but more as a secondary effect of increased liver function. Bilious symptoms, digestive or toxic headaches from hepatic insufficiency, and indigestion may all be helped when Ceanothus is indicated. In addition, Ceanothus will act to mobilize congestion in the lymphatic mesentery that surrounds the intestinal tract.

The despondency and low-grade depression that often accompanies long-term illness may also be relieved by the enhanced liver function that comes with taking this herb. Hemorrhoids and varicosities may become less symptomatic as portal congestion is relieved and pressure is lessened in the venous system of the rectum and lower extremities. Simultaneously, flavonoids and tannins present in the plant function to increase the integrity of vessel walls, further strengthening venous circulation.

A concomitant symptom that often confirms the need for Ceanothus is easy bruising. One young man's capillaries were so fragile that simply running the tip of a fingernail lightly along the skin left a red line that remained for 24 - 72 hours. He had seen several dermatologists who diagnosed dermatography but could offer no treatment for the condition. Fifteen drops of a tincture of Ceanothus taken three times per day completely cleared the underlying etiology of capillary fragility and the symptoms resolved within a few weeks. The patient was able to discontinue the herb after 3 months without relapse.

Ceanothus is mildly antiseptic and may be used as a gargle for tonsillitis, pharyngitis, and canker sores in the mouth. Here it combines well with Echinacea, Hydrastis, Commiphora myrrh, Calendula, Phytolacca, or Baptisia. The plant may also act as an expectorant, when used in formulas for bronchitis and asthma.

Ceanothus has proven to be invaluable in my clinic for the treatment of hemolytic anemia, decreasing the need for transfusions, and reducing splenomegaly. In these cases, I make up a homeopathic preparation from the tincture and administer a 6C potency 3 - 4 times per day in addition to dosing the patient with 15 - 30 drops of tincture 3 times daily.

One patient, a 70-year-old male with severe hemolytic anemia, responded with an increase in both RBC (red blood count) and hematocrit (another indicator of red blood cell concentration in the blood) within three weeks of taking Ceanothus in tincture and potency, as described above. He also reported significant improvement of debilitating fatigue, dizziness, and weakness and was able to begin spacing his regular blood transfusions out for longer and longer periods, much to the astonishment of his hematologist. Ceanothus was the only new treatment he received during that time.

Interestingly, I discovered a study some years later confirming the use of Ceanothus in the 6th potency in combination with tincture for thalassemia patients. The remedy was shown to reduce splenomegaly and increase time between transfusions. Remedies were selected in keeping with classical principles of prescribing the similar medicine.[80]

I would not expect tinctured herb alone without the addition of the potentized low dose homeopathic Ceanothus to be enough for these more pathological cases.

Clinical experience has also shown Ceanothus to be effective at controlling idiopathic thrombocytopenia.

Chamaelirium luteum, Helonias dioica (False Unicorn Root) Liliaceae

Chamaelirium is specific for pelvic stagnation accompanied by a sensation of dragging, heaviness, and fullness in pelvic organs, which are worse during menses. There may be aching in the pelvis, a pushing sensation with menses, and a tendency to prolapse. The symptom of dragging is repeated in the mental emotional sphere where mental dullness, irritability, depression, lack of libido, and low spirited apathy predominate. The patient may be anemic and there may be a sticky leucorrhea. Chamaelirium supports digestive function and increases appetite. It acts as a uterine tonic, and judging from the symptoms that call for its use, the plant is probably more appropriate for uterine laxity than for hypertonicity. It may also act as a diuretic.

Chamaelirium may be used for premenstrual breast tenderness and fibrocystic breast syndrome, but as it is a threatened species, use of Ceanothus for this condition is wiser, as Ceanothus is both highly effective and abundant in nature.

For men, Chamaelirium may be considered for epididymitis, prostatitis and prostatic hypertrophy.

Chamealirium has been listed by United Plant Savers as a threatened species so please use only when specific indications call for it. There are a few farmers beginning to cultivate Chamaelirium and these sources would be preferable to the use of wildcrafted herb.[81] A few drops can be mixed in a formula with other pelvic movers where it will act as a synergist when symptoms reveal it to be specifically indicated. The rhizome is used in medicine.

Foquieria splendens (Ocotillo) Foquieriadaceae

Native to the deserts of the Southwestern United States, ocotillo sends its shoots dramatically up from the earth and straight to the heavens. Unwilling to be hindered on its skyward journey by side roads and detours, this plant does not bother itself with branches, choosing instead to place its leaves directly on the many trunks that spring from a central spot on the earth. In winter, ocotillo dies back so thoroughly one would swear it was nothing more than a bundle of dead branches sticking out of the ground. But come spring, the plant returns strikingly beautiful, with trunks full of green leaves and a sudden burst of red flowers at the towering tips. It reminds us to honor the cycles of life, to balance movement with rest, action with contemplation, and upward surges with downward surrender.

Although I have not used octotillo in this way, it might be a good plant to consider as a spiritual ally when our lives appear to be reduced to a pile of ashes. As it resurrects from appearing dead in winter, so too it may help us resurrect from the ashes of loss and destruction. Not coincidentally, I first met this rising phoenix in Phoenix, Arizona.

This herb is an effective lymph mover and pelvic decongestant and can be considered for any condition in the pelvis where congestion and sluggishness predominate for both men and women. It may, for example, be a useful adjunctive herb for the treatment of benign prostatic hypertrophy in men.

Like Ceanothus, ocotillo stimulates portal circulation in the liver. As a lymphatic it is useful for treating tonsillitis, where it can be dosed whenever acute or chronic lymphatic stagnation presents.

Patients who seem scattered, running in many directions, without focus or time for contemplation, may be well served by ocotillo. Similarly, those folks who find themselves unable to get moving may discover a little more energy and motivation as circulation is mobilized, stagnant lymph is released, and liver function is enhanced. The plant encourages us to move from our center, without losing ourselves or dissipating our energy.[82]

The bark is used in medicine. It is another plant to be used judiciously, and is a protected species in the state of Arizona. Constituents include glucosides and resins.

Gossypium herbaceum, G. thurberi (Cotton Root Bark) Malvaceae

Historically, the fresh inner root bark of the cotton plant was used by African-American slaves in the old south as an abortifacient. Although I do not have information about dosing for this purpose, the plant was reputed to be very effective in this regard. Gossypium is useful as an emmenogogue for slow to start, sluggish menses with a sensation of dragging in the pelvis and concomitant dull low back pain or discomfort. It tonifies the uterine muscle and may prove useful in bringing the postpartum uterus back to normal size. Moore tells us that the plant works synergistically with the body's endogenous oxytocin to induce or speed up labor in cases where pitocin is being considered. Post partum it may also be considered as a galactogogue.

Presence of astringent tannins imply a likely anti-hemorrhagic effect for excessive menstrual or post partum bleeding and the recent scientific literature suggests that the use of Gossypium may be of aid in treating breast cancer.[83] Other constituents include a resin and essential oils.

Leonurus cardiaca (Motherwort) Labiatae

As a pelvic herb, Leonurus acts as an emmenogogue when menses are sluggish in starting or delayed in onset. As a uterine tonic and anti-spasmodic nervine, it is useful for treating menstrual cramping, especially when associated with stagnant menses. It is also helpful in alleviating premenstrual tension, water retention, and menopausal symptoms.

Constituents in leonurus include flavonoids, glycosides, and several alkaloids. The leaves are used in medicine.

Nuphar luteum, Nypmhaea odorata (Yellow/White Pond Lily) Nymphaceae

Pond lily is very specific for inflammatory conditions in the pelvis and is contraindicated when congestion is of a cold, non-inflammatory nature, as is seen with uterine fibroids. Pelvic decongestant properties combine with the plant's cooling actions to make pond lily helpful in treating urinary tract inflammation, acute flare-ups of interstitial cystitis, urethritis, and prostatitis. Hydrocele, epididymitis, leucorrhea, bacterial vaginosis with acute irritation of mucous membranes of the vagina, mid cycle ovarian pain, ruptured ovarian cysts, acute pelvic inflammatory disease, and other acute inflammatory conditions of pelvic organs may all be helped by the addition of pond lily. It is also indicated for hot inflammatory conditions of the gastro-intestinal tract such as colitis and gastritis. Pains, when present, tend to be sharp in quality, and another herb should be considered if the patient describes their pain as dull and achy.

The plant's astringency helps tighten up mucous membrane surfaces when there is too copious a discharge, making it useful for the treatment of leucorrhea. Here it is an excellent medicine when taken internally, because it also keeps circulation and lymph flowing through the pelvis, thereby addressing, at least in part, the underlying cause. Pond lily is effective for stimulating lymphatics throughout the body.

Constituents include alkaloids, phytosterols, mucilage, tannins, and flavonoids and one species of Nymphaea has been shown in research to possess anti-oxidant activity due to the presence of a significant number of flavonoids.[84,85] Another species, Nymphaea stellata, used in Ayurvedic medicine, has been shown to be hepato-protective.[86]

Botanically, these plants are related to the much-revered East Indian lotus, sacred to Hindu tradition. The roots of pond lily used for medicine must be dug from the depths of muddy, slimy ponds. The beautiful lotus or pond lily that rests so peacefully on the surface of the water and draws its sustenance from the murky depths below reminds us that the initiation into enlightenment draws its nourishment from our willingness to dive into the shadowy depths of the soul, often a messy and painful process. An old alchemical saying repeats the message of the pond lily when it states,

"For a tree's branches to reach to heaven, its roots must reach to hell."

In the end, these plants remind us that if we are willing to persevere, we too may learn to draw sustenance from the darker side of life until at last we are able to rise to the surface, floating peacefully in the light, and glowing with a wise beauty that radiates out to bless others who cross our paths. In the meantime, nature has blessed us with pond lily and lotus to aid us on this journey.

Turnera aphrodesiatica/diffusa (Damiana) Turneraceae

Damiana is a hormonal, digestive, and central nervous system tonic. It is a good pelvic decongestant herb to consider for chronic urinary irritation, as with interstitial cystitis, or when there is a tendency to repeated urinary tract infections.

Although primarily used for treating pelvic congestion in men, damiana may be used for women with dysmenorrhea, leucorrhea due to pelvic stagnation, or amenorrhea. For men it earns its species name of aphrodesiatica by virtue of its activity as a reproductive and sexual tonic where it combines well with Smilax, Catuaba and Ptychopetalum for erectile dysfunction. Pedicularis, an excellent musculo-skeletal nervine is also reputed to help with erectile dysfunction.[87] There is some thought that damiana's flavonoid content may be contributing to its ability to resurrect waning sexual function, as similar flavonoids have been isolated from yohimbe, a more commonly known herb that has been used in the treatment of erectile dysfunction. Damiana may also be used to diminish prostatic congestion common to benign prostatic hypertrophy.

As a nervine, damiana is uplifting, invigorating, and antidepressant.

Damiana has anti-inflammatory activity due at least in part to the presence of flavonoids. Traditional use in Brazil, where the plant is indigenous, includes treatment of gastric ulcer, an application which has been validated in animal studies.[88] The plant also has some astringent qualities.

Some authors suggest this herb can be depleting if used over too long a time. I have not noticed this effect using smaller doses in a larger formula, but the herb does contain some caffeine.

Constituents include arbutin, flavonoids, terpenoids, saccharides, phenolics, caffeine, and an essential oil. The leaves are used in medicine.

Thuja occidentalis, T. plicata (Western Cedar) Pinaceae

The needles of cedar trees used in medicine, although not highly toxic, are dose sensitive and should be administered with respect. Lower doses are tonic and stimulate function of tissues where laxity is present, whereas higher doses can be over stimulating to tissues, causing irritation to mucosal tissues. 10 - 30 drops of a 1:0.9 fresh liquid extract may be given up to four times per day. (Tilgner) Dr. Bastyr used 3 drops of tincture several times throughout the day for cystitis (Mitchell).

Constituents include bitter compounds, a glucoside, and essential oils, including thujone.

Thuja is anti-bacterial, anti-viral and anti-fungal. As a mucous membrane tonic and anti-microbial it has been used for respiratory infections and bladder infections. For the former, it is perhaps best inhaled in a steam, delivering the antiseptic essential oils directly to the site of infection. Thuja also acts as a tonic and stimulant to kidney and digestive function.

Thuja is useful as a reproductive tonic in cases of atony. For women with amenorrhea it may help act as an emmenogogue. It is one of the main ingredients in the "vag packs" utilized by naturopathic physicians for cervical dysplasia, HPV infections, bacterial vaginosis, chronic pelvic inflammatory disease and pelvic congestion. These packs, available from Eclectic Institute in Sandy, Oregon, contain a mixture of herbs and mineral salts. The pack is placed into the vaginal vault overnight for local application to the cervix where it acts as a drawing poultice to aid in the extraction of toxins from the pelvic cavity.

As a pelvic decongestant and disinfectant, Thuja is well indicated for urinary incontinence due to weak bladder muscles. It can be of help for stress incontinence in women or in the dribbling of urine associated with benign prostatic hypertrophy. It is useful for weakness of the bladder in either gender and should also be considered for men suffering with chronic prostatitis. When combined with Zea mays and Hypericum perforatum, it has served well for bladder weakness during or after menopause.

For children it has been used in the treatment of nocturnal enuresis (bedwetting) where it may be combined with Belladonna. (Felter) Thuja may act as a diuretic, stimulant, or disinfectant in the urinary tract.

Although the mental emotional picture need not be present to prescribe an herb, the person who will be most helped by this plant may be closed, suspicious, suppressed, have a tendency to develop warts or report a history of sexually transmitted diseases. There may be a sense of separateness from themselves or from others. Homeopathically it is one of the main remedies for treating symptoms from over vaccination when the patient's personality fits the picture just described.

Thuja essential oil has some reputation for treating warts when applied topically. I have not seen it be all that useful alone, but other practitioners swear by it. I do find that when Thuja essential oil is used to wet down a bit of powdered Sanguinaria canadensis (bloodroot) and applied to a wart, covered, and left overnight for several nights, the wart generally begins to disintegrate in short order. Although it may not work as quickly, a tincture of Sanguinaria mixed with the Thuja essential oil will also eradicate the wort when powdered Sanguinaria is hard to come by.

Internal use of an anti-viral formula addresses immune issues that predispose to the formation of warts and is an indispensible addition to the topical treatment. Such a formula might include Thuja spp., Hypericum perforatum (St. John's Wort,) Ligusticum porteri (osha), Lomatium dissectum (lomatium), Melissa officinalis (lemon balm), Glycerrhiza glabra (licorice root) and should be given at doses of 30 - 60 drops 3 - 4 times daily. Hypericum should be included for genital warts (HPV) as it is spiritually protective to the pelvic and genital area as well as anti-viral.

The essential oil of Thuja has also been used as a topical treatment for tinea (ringworm) infections of the skin.

In large doses Thuja acts as an irritant to the gastro-intestinal tract, kidneys and lungs. It can produce violent symptoms in the digestive tract with vomiting, nausea, and intestinal cramping. Heart rate may be increased. Urinary retention, renal damage, and seizures are late signs. The presence of the essential oil thujone is the constituent most responsible for toxicity. The oil is not easily soluble in water making the tea safer and still quite efficacious.

Mitchella repens (Partridge Berry) Rubiaceae

Mitchella is specific for uterine congestion with atony and overly lax muscles. There may be hemorrhage, bright red bleeding, dysmenorrhea, or uterine congestion accompanied by achiness in the low back.

As an astringent, it has been used for excessive menstrual bleeding and postpartum hemorrhage. In pregnancy, Mitchella finds use as a preventative in threatened miscarriage of later pregnancy and is commonly used as a partus preparator in the third trimester. It may be safely used throughout lactation as well.

For men Mitchella should be considered for prostatitis and the symptoms of dysuria associated with benign prostatic hypertrophy. Mitchella has nervine properties that bring relief to irritability and anxiety.

One of the common names, "squaw vine," draws from a derogatory label for Native American women and its use is discouraged for that reason. The leaves or entire above ground parts of the plant are used in medicine.

Raspberry Leaf (Rubus spp.) Rosaceae

When taken as a tea throughout the month, raspberry leaf works well as a uterine tonic for dysmenorrhea where it acts to soothe spasmodic uterine muscles or, conversely, to tone lax boggy muscles. Raspberry improves pelvic circulation and like so many members of the rose family, acts as an astringent in cases where excessive menstrual bleeding is an issue.

Pulsatilla (Anemone spp.) Ranunculaceae

In spite of a widespread notion that Pulsatilla is an herb for women, Eclectic prescribers of the early twentieth century often used it for prostatitis, benign prostatic hypertrophy, and other disorders of the male reproductive tract. It is best prescribed on specific indications and will serve well in the mild, eager to please male, or the tough guy secretly hiding a vulnerable little boy. Pulsatilla is also indicated for epididymitis, spermatorrhea, urethral irritation, and orchitis with dark red swelling and exquisite sensitivity of the testicles.

For women, Pulsatilla will aid with delayed, scanty, or suppressed menses, especially when due to stress, nervous exhaustion, or from getting her feet cold and wet. When taken all month long, it acts as a uterine tonic for the treatment of dysmenorrhea. A sensation of weakness and fullness in low back and hips may accompany pelvic symptoms.

Ovarian symptoms include neuralgia, with a dull, nagging, achy pain that can turn more violent if allowed to persist untreated. Pelvic inflammation or endometriosis may be present.

Leucorrhea when present will be bland, thick, white or yellowish in character while premenstrual symptoms include headaches, irritability, depression, and weepiness.

Pulsatilla is an important hepatic and digestive herb where it is particularly helpful if symptoms of indigestion occur after indulgence in rich creamy foods, pastries or fatty foods. There may be bilious headaches after fatty foods. The tongue may have a greasy coat and there may be diarrhea alternating with constipation.

The patient generally presents as mild, yielding, and eager to please often with a tendency to weep, sometimes without knowing why. Gloominess, with timidity and fearfulness are common symptoms. Irritability, despondency, depression, or sadness may accompany physical symptoms. Anxiety is a significant complaint that may present with nervous exhaustion, debility, insomnia and restlessness as part of the picture. There is a general pattern of disempowerment coupled with a desire for affection and fear of abandonment.

Pulsatilla should also be considered for nervousness due to abuse of tobacco.

Venous congestions, varicosities, and hemorrhoids reflect liver congestion and the general tendency to weakness in vessels. Pale women with anemia who complain of feeling chilly and weak also respond well to this plant.

Pulsatilla acts as a cardiac tonic where it is used for functional heart palpitations, anxiety induced tachycardia, dyspnea, and a pulse that is weak and feeble. The herb acts to slow and strengthen the heart and respiration, increase circulation to the central nervous system, and increase peripheral circulation.

The herb has been used internally for glaucoma, iritis, scleritis and cataracts. There may be a deep seated heavy pain in the globe of the eye. It has also been used in the treatment of conjunctivitis. Homeopathic preparations of the plant are very effective for acute conjunctivitis in patients of any age. I have almost never seen it fail for these cases.

Discharges tend to be bland, thick, yellow or white, but usually there is a tendency to dryness and thirstlessness.

While the plant is ant-inflammatory in therapeutic doses, excessive doses can manifest as gastroentertitis with burning pains in mouth and throat, abdominal pain, nausea, vomiting, and bloody diarrhea. Paralysis, sensory and motor nerve depression, convulsions, coma and death are a result of toxicity to the nervous system. Cardiac symptoms of overdose include arrythymias, feeble pulse, bradycardia, and dyspnea. The plant is contraindicated in bradycardia and acute gastro-intestinal inflammation. It is one of the top remedies to treat gastritis and gastro-esophageal reflux when used homeopathically.

Dosage of 1:2 fresh whole plant tincture should not exceed 5-10 drops three times per day. (Tilgner) Preparations must be made from fresh plant material to be effective.

Serenoa repens (Saw Palmetto) Palmaceae

Serenoa is an excellent pelvic decongestant, used primarily for treating conditions affecting the male reproductive tract, although it is used in certain situations for women as well. The plant has become a popular over the counter remedy for treating symptoms of benign prostatic hypertrophy (BPH) in older men, where it is specifically indicated when urination is difficult, with dribbling. In addition to androgen modulation and inhibition of 5-alpha reductase,[89] Serenoa acts as a tonic to the musculature of the urinary bladder, thereby encouraging more complete emptying of the bladder. Several of the plant's free fatty acids contribute to block the enzymatic conversion of testosterone to dihydro-testosterone and interfere with the ability of dihyro-testosterone to bind to cell receptor sites in affected organs.[90]

Serenoa should also be considered in the treatment of prostatitis, epididymitis, urethritis, orchalgia, and orchitits. It may help with low or absent libido and is an important nutritive tonic whenever erectile dysfunction is an issue, although it has been my experience that there are other herbs that act more powerfully in this regard.

As a nourishing tonic for the urinary tract, Serenoa has found use in enuresis of children, recurrent or chronic urinary tract infections, and interstitial cystitis. Anti-spasmodic actions help with urinary tenesmus, although pelvic pain that is dull and aching is not a contraindication.

Anti-inflammatory activity contributes to the herb's anti-spasmodic, alterative, and nutritive qualities. Serenoa enhances digestive function, improving appetite and assimilation, soothes the nervous system, and may help in respiratory complaints where it acts as an expectorant.

For women, Serenoa has recently found popularity in the treatment of polycystic ovarian syndrome, where it's ability to modulate androgen metabolism may help mitigate effects of excess androgen production in the body. It has also been used for inflammation of the ovaries, dull aching pain in the ovaries, and leucorrhea due to laxity of the uterine muscle.

Constituents include several free fatty acids, lauric acid, myristic acid, palmitic acid, linoleic acid, and oleic acid. Phytosterols, specifically beta sitosterol, monoglycerides and free fatty alcohols are also present.

The dried berries are hard enough to break the average blender, so take care if you decide to prepare an extract yourself. The berries may be decocted using 1 - 2 teaspoons for each cup of water, or a tincture of 1:2.5 strength may be administered at 15 - 60 drops up to 4 times daily.

Uterine Tonics

Alchemilla vulgaris (Lady's Mantle)
Angelica sinensis (Chinese Angelica)
Caulophyllum thalictroides (Blue Cohosh)
Mitchella repens (Partridge Berry)
Rubus idaeus (Raspberry Leaf)

Specific to Ovaries

Caulophylum thalistroides (Blue Cohosh)
Anemone vulgaris, A. pratensis (Pulsatilla)
Serenoa repens (Saw Pametto) PCOS
Ceanothus spp. (Red Root, Wild Lilac) specific for cysts

Anti-Hemorrhagics

Achillea millefolium (Yarrow)
Alchemilla vulgaris (Lady's Mantle)
Capsella bursa-pastorius (Shepherd's Purse)
Ceanothus spp. (Red Root, Wild Lilac)
Anemone spp. (Pulsatilla)
Rubus idaeus (Raspberry Leaf)

Inflammation (PID)

Achillea milefolium (Yarrow)
Caulophyllum thalictroides (Blue Cohosh)
Cimicifuga/Actea racemosa (Black Cohosh)
Nuphar/Nymphaea spp. (Pond Lilies)

Hormonal Modulation

Angelica sinensis (Chinese Angelica)
Arctium lappa (Burdock Root)
Asparagus racemosa (Shatavari)
Cimicifuga/Actea racemosa (Black Cohosh)
Dioscorea villosa (Wild Yam)
Foeniculum vulgare (Fennel)
Glycerrhiza glabra (Licorice Root)
Medicago sativa (Alfalfa)
Mitchella repens (Partridge Berry)
Serenoa repens (Saw Palmetto)
Smilax ornata (Sarsaparilla)
Taraxacum officinalis (Dandelion)
Urtica dioica root (Nettle Root)
Vitex agnus-castus (Chaste Tree Berry)

Prostate/Epididymis/Testes

Chamelirium lutem/Helonias dioica (False Unicorn Root)
Cimicifuga/Actea racemosa (Black Cohosh)
Foqueria splendens (Ocotillo)
Anemone spp. (Pulsatilla)
Pygeum africana (Pygeum)
Serenoa (Saw Palmetto)
Thuja plicata/occidentalis (Western Red Cedar)
Turnera aphrodisiatica (Damiana)

Chapter 12
Menarche and Moontime

"Women are hope. That is sort of how we look at women... Women have the ability to reproduce, and so a woman always has that hope instilled within her. So, that was the premise to preventing, you know, like abuses of women sexually, emotionally, and physically, whatever, because you would jeopardize that hope."

Schwartz, Maureen Trudelle, Molded in Image of Changing Women: Navajo Views on the Human Body and Personhood, University of Arizona Press, Tucson, 1997, pp. 184-185 (quoting Sunny Dooley, Gallup, NM, 1992)

ALTHOUGH MODERN HOLISTIC HEALING stresses the importance of treating each patient as a whole being, there is still a vast abyss to be bridged in the area of gynecology and women's reproductive health with regards to the spiritual aspects of being incarnate in a female body.

For women, the inner worlds of emotional, intuitive and mystical experience have a doorway in the physical realm of the menstrual cycle, from the earliest prepubescent awakenings of menarche, through every menstrual cycle and precious pregnancy we carry, into the final transition of menopause. Our cycles keep us intimately connected to the earth, providing us with an untold abundance of opportunity for spiritual unfolding that is grounded in the natural processes of our bodies.

Traditional earth-honoring cultures throughout the world have always honored women's monthly blood flow as a time of power, when intuitive abilities are heightened and the veil between everyday reality and the world of Spirit is thinned. In these communities, time is set aside to take advantage of the increased sensitivity that enhances introspection and spiritual practice. The traditional Moon Lodge or the Red Tent creates a protected ritual space for women to experience the intuitive power of Moontime, as well as process the strong feelings that often emerge with the onset of menses. The increased sensitivity and emotional awareness that accompanies this time of month is viewed as a gift that enables women to connect to the world of Spirit more readily. When women are regularly deprived of the space needed for contemplation and renewal, irritability, and a snappish insistence on being left alone often ensues. The inner vitality of the women is demanding that the needs of her spirit be met.

Because women are naturally more open just before and during menses, there is also more sensitivity to external negativity in the environment. The Moon Lodge offers women protection as well as a time of rest. In many cultures, women are not even allowed to cook at this time, which not only gives the women a much needed break, but also offers the rest of the community an opportunity to ritually honor the uterine blood that once nourished and birthed us all through feeding the women in Moon Lodge.

The irritability and desire to be left alone that so many women feel just before and during menses is symptomatic of our need for solitude during a time that is meant for contemplation and renewal. Even physical symptoms will be healed more readily if spiritual needs are fulfilled.

Our modern world no longer has the wisdom to honor and flow with the cycles of nature, thus we do not generally have the sense to honor the natural cycles of our bodies. Electric lights allow us to stay up hours after sunset, and instead of slowing down in the dark of winter and taking time for introspection, we continue our frenzied pace of doing, doing, doing. Despite these impediments in consciousness and culture, women can still do much to honor their Sacred Time of Bleeding. Simply taking more time to rest, meditate, go within, and process the feelings and intuitive experiences that emerge during the flow can be very powerful. Doing so is, in fact, the only real cure I have ever seen for menstrual cramps.

"...young women are acknowledged to have a unique power while experiencing their first and second menstrual periods."

Schwartz, Maureen Trudelle, Molded in the Image of Changing Woman: Navajo Views on the Human Body and Personhood, University of Arizona Press, Tucson, 1997, p. 175

In healthy Indigenous cultures puberty ceremonies are traditional for young men as well as young women. These ceremonies include teachings that bring spiritual connection, protection, health, and blessings to young people which will continue to guide them throughout their adult lives. While the industrialized world tends to joke about the "raging hormones" of adolescence, more earth-centered cultures recognize that sacred life generating forces are incarnating into us as we enter adulthood. What we recognize as hormonal shifts, wiser cultures acknowledge as the power to bring forth life. Such vital energy is treasured, nourished and guided as young people are given tools to work with the new, unfamiliar forces that begin to surge through their bodies, thus creating a container for newly emerging life giving powers to be integrated in ways that guide away from confusion, disrespect and violence. These coming of age rituals enhance the lives of not only each individual teen, but the entire community in which they live. Contrast this with industrialized society where young people are largely misunderstood, rejected, or ridiculed as "crazy teenagers" by a culture whose ritual coming of age ceremonies have been lost through generations of oppression and genocide.

Our loss of connection to all that is sacred in nature has resulted in a cultural travesty that directly affects our health. The ensuing lack of ritual honoring of important physical life transitions has a significant impact on our physical well-being. Among the Navajo it was observed that when Native American children were taken from their families and placed into boarding schools, the young girls who entered menarche while away at school, and hence missed their coming of age ceremony, were more prone in the ensuing years to experience difficulties with reproductive health.[91]

Many parents today are beginning to recognize the importance of honoring the transition from childhood to adulthood, by gathering tools to recreate what was lost and offer their own children something they may never have had themselves. This rebirth of ceremonial celebration offers hope for future generations and all people everywhere.

What can be more sacred than the distinctly female power of pregnancy and childbirth, the extraordinary process of building, carrying, nourishing, and birthing new life? When we women labor to usher life onto the earth from the spirit world, our consciousness is altered rendering us once again more receptive to spiritual realms. If pregnant women know the potential for spiritual connection is inherent in the physical experience of giving birth, an opportunity becomes available to deepen the experience of labor and delivery, as the woman's spirit reaches across the divide to welcome a new soul from the spirit world and guide him or her into incarnation in a physical body.

One woman, who had a very difficult time during the birth of her first child, reported seeing angels in the room on delivering her next. She played sacred songs throughout her second labor and welcomed the experience as a spiritual adventure, full of joy and celebration.

Menopause offers women yet another opportunity to honor the changes flowing through these earth bodies during the transition from mothering years to elder. If we are willing and able to go within to contemplate and follow the flow of our emotions and intuition we may discover an opportunity to welcome the wisdom that is literally being shapeshifted into our whole beings. Surges of power meld into us as hot flashes or sudden irritability arise inviting us to integrate the fire and claim a new level of energy that will strengthen our elder years. Plenty of quiet time, preferably in nature, nourishes the journey from one phase of life to the next.

While herbs and other natural therapies are integral to helping us on the road to becoming and staying healthy, they are only our helpers along the way. We do our green growing relatives a great disservice if we do not do our part by reclaiming, celebrating, and loving our beautiful female bodies in all their various shapes and sizes.

Introductory Comments

A formula of pelvic decongestant herbs offers an important foundation for treating conditions of both male and female reproductive tracts. For women, problems such as dysmenorrhea, mid cycle ovarian discomfort (Mettelschmirtz), uterine fibroids, cervical dysplasia, dysfunctional uterine bleeding, ovarian cysts, endometriosis, pelvic inflammation, and bacterial vaginosis are a few of the conditions that are aggravated or caused by pelvic stagnation. Irregular menses, amenorrhea, meno-metrorrhagia, and polycystic ovarian syndrome will also respond to the addition of pelvic moving herbs to a constitutional treatment plan. Most conditions affecting reproductive organs will heal more readily if the liver and adrenal glands are nourished and supported to correct underlying hormonal imbalances. Thyroid function should also be assessed and treated as necessary.

Dysmenorrhea

"Your blood is sacred and speaks of your womanliness. Be proud of your time. It is not the 'curse' as you white women call it."

Andrews, Lynn V., Flight of the Seventh Moon, The Teachings of the Shields, Harper and Row, 1984, p 77

Experience in clinic has shown that women who are struggling with dysmenorrhea or PMS do not fully benefit from naturopathic therapies until they are able to honor each monthly flow by taking whatever time and space is needed to honor the opportunities for sacred connection and wholeness that each monthly cycle offers. After learning the value of introspection during menstrual flow, several women have reported to me that they notice a shift in cramping pain when they take time away for contemplation, rest, and regeneration. Cramps increase when these women try to be in their intellectual or active selves, only to disappear once they follow the pain inward for contemplation, meditation, or a simple rejuvenating nap.

Naturopathic treatment of acute menstrual pain can be initiated with an individual herb or a combination of any of the following plants.

Viburnum opulus (cramp bark)

Viburnum can be dosed aggressively, taking 1 teaspoon every one to two hours or 15 drops every 15 minutes as needed. (Tilgner).

Dioscorea villosa (wild yam)

Eschscholzia californica (California poppy)

These two herbs can be dosed 60 drops, 4 times per day, although smaller doses taken more frequently may be more effective.

When combining these herbs together, Viburnum should make up at least half of the formula, with equal parts of the other two herbs mixed in.

Uterine tonics such as raspberry leaf, Angelica sinensis, Caulophyllum, Mitchella repens, or Actea should be taken throughout the month. A supplement of calcium, magnesium and Vitamin D may also be helpful.

Do not assume a patient has adequate vitamin D levels, regardless of how much time they spend in the sun. For whatever reason, clinicians are finding deficiencies of this vitamin in astonishingly high numbers. If current serum levels of vitamin D are unavailable, it is generally safe to take 1500-2000 I.U. daily. Adequate blood levels of vitamin D are essential for calcium to be taken into the cells.

Mag phos 6X can be taken for menstrual cramps every two hours along with the herbal formula created for the acute symptoms. If the 6X Mag Phos proves ineffective, a 30C may be given every 4 hours or a 200C every 4 to 8 hours.

Atropa belladonna (Belladonna)

In cases of severe dysmenorrhea that are not relieved by the previous applications, a tincture of Atropa belladonna, (1:10 dry herb) is invariably effective. Twenty-five (25) drops of Belladonna tincture should be mixed with enough water to equal a total volume of 4 ounces. This diluted solution may be given at doses of one teaspoonful every 1 - 2 hours as needed. In more severe cramping, a teaspoonful may be repeated every 15 minutes for 3 - 4 doses to start, moving to the every 1 - 2 hour schedule after that. A potent and highly toxic plant, Belladonna should be used with caution. No more than 24 teaspoons should be taken over a 24 hour period. Belladonna tincture is also highly effective for the intestinal spasm that often accompanies inflammatory bowel disease.

Symptoms of overdose of belladonna include dry mouth, inability to perspire, flushed face, tachycardia, hyperpyrexia (increased temperature), headache, dilated pupils, dryness, hoarseness and constriction in throat, constipation, urinary retention, difficulty breathing, coma and death.

PMS/Premenstrual Syndrome

There is within each of us, a compelling urge that rises from the depths of our souls to lead us to wholeness. When we attempt to ignore, suppress, or subvert this drive for unity, we block the soul's sincere desire to move us forward. Thus, if we do not consciously strive to integrate the inward surges of vitality that our souls long to bring to us, these parts of our humanity will often express unconsciously, in ways that are often not as constructive as a more conscious, self-accepting expression might be.

The moodiness and irritability that many women complain of as their moontime approaches is often an attempt by a deeper spiritual self to get the much needed space that a traditional Moon Lodge offers for inward reflection, processing, revitalization, and spiritual practice. When strong, seemingly irrational emotions arise at Moontime, women should be encouraged to honor the process even if feelings seem extreme. The heart cares little for the opinions of the cerebral cortex in such matters and much wisdom can be gained by sitting with our emotions in an open-hearted and compassionate way. Inviting our tears, anxieties, irritability, and resentments in by conversing or journaling with feelings is generally more productive than judging and suppressing unpleasant emotions, which rarely works in any case.

Instead of rejecting emotions, it may be more helpful to imagine welcoming a difficult emotion in for a cup of tea and initiating dialogue with questions such as

"How are you here to serve me?"

"What do you need?"

When answers bring up challenging or unpleasant issues, dialogue can be continued with responses such as

"That scares me, I could never do that."

"I don't understand. Tell me more."

This process should be continued until the emotion eases or there are no more answers. The first part of the dialogue will often bring up information that is already apparent or easily accessible to consciousness. Continued dialogue allows for deeper connection, bringing more revealing, and potentially transformative insights from the unconscious.

Although it is unfortunately impractical for the modern woman to retreat to a Moon Lodge for a few days during her blood flow, we can encourage women to take extra time to rest and regenerate. Meditative techniques can be utilized to replace negative feelings women may carry about their reproductive organs with love and deep appreciation for the Beauty of the female form, while receptivity to the spiritual power that naturally flows with Moontime offers subtle opportunities for integrating wisdom and enhancing intuition.

Naturopathic therapies can ease the emotional and spiritual integration process, lightening the burden by clearing liver congestion, nourishing overstressed adrenals and nervous systems, and clearing stagnation. Flower essences and homeopathy are particularly helpful when emotional symptoms predominate while assessing liver, thyroid, and adrenal health is essential for any condition related to reproductive organs and hormone balance. All of these therapies bring relief to emotional turmoil and ease physical symptoms, not by suppressing or robbing the woman of her process, but by removing obstacles, clearing the way, and hastening the process along, making integration and consciousness more easily accessible.

Needless to say establishing a good foundation for health is vital in all these cases, as with anything we treat.

Premenstrual, Toxic, and Migraine Headaches

The female reproductive hormones estrogen and progesterone released by the ovaries during each monthly cycle need to be processed and cleared as each cycle ends and menses begin. If the liver is congested with a backlog of environmental toxins, hormones may not get broken down as efficiently. Conversely, the need to break down normal circulating hormones at the end of each cycle may mean toxins don't get cleared as efficiently in an already overloaded liver. For this reason, headaches that occur before or during the menstrual cycle are often a result of suboptimal liver function and can therefore generally be considered toxic headaches. Poor diet, food sensitivities, exogenous toxins, or liver/gall bladder stagnation can all contribute to liver congestion. Hormone imbalances can often be corrected when liver stagnation is addressed. Maintaining open and efficient emunctories (channels of elimination) is essential to discharge accumulated toxins. Toxic or "sick" headaches, as they are sometimes called, can sometimes be differentiated from tension headaches by their timing in relationship to the menstrual cycle, digestive upset, food indiscretions, or exposure to environmental toxins. Not infrequently, toxic headaches will be accompanied by digestive symptoms, such as low appetite, nausea, and possibly vomiting.

Tension headaches, which are different from migraines, digestive, or premenstrual headaches, respond well to formulas outlined earlier for musculo-skeletal spasm.

The following herbal formula can be given continuously throughout the month to tone liver and digestive function and prevent congestive premenstrual headaches while nutritional and constitutional issues are being corrected. Migraine headaches will also respond to this formula of herbs.

Tanacetum parthenim (Feverfew) ....5 drams
Lavandula officinalis (Lavender) ....2 drams
Zinginber officianale (Ginger) ....1 dram

The herbs are best given 10 - 15 minutes before meals as the bitters in the feverfew and lavender stimulate digestion and liver function. The ginger in the formula acts as a warming, circulatory stimulant and digestive carminative as well as an anti-inflammatory synergist. The lavender, in addition to being indicated for toxic headaches and migraines, is protective and calming to the nervous system, while the feverfew moves stagnant liver energy, promotes detoxification, and acts as an anti-inflammatory peripheral vasodilator, bringing congestion down from the head by dilating peripheral blood vessels.

For headache prevention and reducing frequency and severity of headaches, the formula may be given at doses of 15 - 60 drops, three times per day throughout the month. A lower dose of 15 - 30 drops is usually adequate except in cases where headaches are very frequent or severe.

At the first sign of a headache, the patient should dose the formula at 5 to 30 drops every 2 hours as needed. The herbs may be repeated as often as every 10 - 15 minutes for the first 3 - 4 doses to hasten the process. The key to repetitive dosing is to have the patient follow the symptoms, and adjust the dose accordingly, but in most cases a dose every 1 - 2 hours is sufficient.

Herbs for headaches work best when taken at the very first sign of pain, in which case one or two doses are usually sufficient. Continued aggressive dosing is generally only needed if the headache is well underway by the time the patient initiates treatment with herbs. If the acute headache is already severe, patients may experience some purging with vomiting and diarrhea. This is probably the work of the feverfew and while the ginger does allay nausea, it will not suppress it if the patient needs the discharge. As long as the feverfew is helping the pain, I instruct the patient to keep dosing as needed. Vomiting is often present with sick headaches even without the herbs, as the body attempts to rid itself of toxic material. Purging only occurs when the headache is already quite severe. Patients whose vitality is weak should not be allowed to purge and obviously prolonged or excessive purging is inappropriate for any patient. These patients should be watched closely and monitored for signs of dehydration or electrolyte imbalance.

The personality of feverfew is that of a strong, no-nonsense, warrior, who charges in to do battle with toxins that stand in the way of vibrant health. Liver and digestive fires gear up, and toxins are history. The only trouble is, if a patient is well into the headache by the time they begin the herb feverfew's warrior cleansing process can leave them feeling pretty ragged, even without any vomiting or diarrhea. That feverfew has won the battle, the headache is gone, but the poor patient's battle-worn nervous system leaves them feeling wasted. Used alone, feverfew can be depleting and hard on the nervous system when taken in doses large enough to alleviate a severe headache.

The addition of lavender, another bitter digestive herb used in treating migraine and toxic headaches, adds nervine actions that soothe and protect the nervous system. This gentle, strong grandmother wisely balances feverfew's fiery male energy, supporting him in battle, but protecting and nourishing the nervous system, thereby preventing the post-war nervous exhaustion that is sometimes seen when feverfew is used alone. The war still happens, but the patient no longer has to experience it. They just feel better.

In acute cases, a hot foot bath with cold applications to the head should accompany the herbal treatment. Have the patient boil a kettle of water to keep at hand. A bucket should be filled with water as hot as is comfortably tolerated, and feet immersed to above the ankles. The kettle of boiled water is kept at hand to add to the footbath as the water cools. Be sure to tell the patient to remove their feet from the bucket before adding more hot water! A bowl with ice water and 2 washcloths is also kept nearby. The patient applies the cold washcloth anywhere on the head that feels good to them, although occiput, vertex, and frontal areas are usually most effective. As one cloth is warmed by the body, it is replaced by the other washcloth so that the cold applications are maintained.

This treatment usually brings relief within 20 minutes, especially when combined with the herbs. Ideally the patient is wrapped in wool blankets with an attendant available to change the cold applications and add more hot water to the footbath, as this enhances elimination through sweating and keeps the hands warm, further encouraging congestion to exit the cranium and descend into the periphery. Powdered ginger may be added to the hot foot bath for increased efficacy.

For the patient who wakes with headaches, the warming sock treatment as described in Chapter II can be instituted and is often efficacious at preventing their occurrence. The socks will be dry by morning as the body circulates blood down from the cranium to warm the feet, thus drawing congestion out of the head. The warming socks should be started a few nights before the expected headache.

Assessing and treating any cranial or spinal fixations is also important any time a patient presents with a tendency to headaches.

Case

A 32 year old single mother reported to clinic with significant fatigue, severe insomnia, and daily headaches that became excruciating a few days before the onset of menses. These symptoms had plagued her for years. Trudging through life with dogged determination, she was overly responsible and worked hard to keep a roof over her head and feed her family of three young children. Despite her constant pain and a sense of inner torment, she was able to put on a cheerful face to the world. Her childhood had been oppressive and abusive leaving her emotionally repressed and plagued by guilt.

Interestingly, a visit to her house revealed a yard full of feverfew and agrimony, the two plants most specific for her condition. I showed her how to make a tincture of the feverfew and encouraged her to dry the agrimony for use in tea to help with the feelings of torment. In addition to the herbs, she was given homeopathic Carcinosin in an LM potency and changes were made to her diet. She was also given a tincture of lavender to mix with feverfew in a ratio of 3 parts lavender to 5 parts feverfew, which she then took in doses of 15 drops three times per day. At the first sign of headache she was instructed to take extra doses of 15 drops every 15 minutes to every 2 hours as needed.

Although the dietary modifications and much needed detoxification protocols that were instituted for her took time, she began to feel a shift in the headaches almost immediately with the herbs. A supportive adrenal formula was included with 7 parts of Uncaria tomentosa and 1 part Oplopanax horridum and was dosed at 60 drops 3 times daily.

The homeopathic remedy had a profound effect on her insomnia as well as helping her emotionally and constitutionally. In a short time, the daily headaches disappeared with her only headaches occurring just prior to menses. After several months of treatment, the feverfew and lavender lost their effectiveness, at which time, Cimicifuga 15 drops 3 times per day all month proved most helpful for preventing the headaches associated with menses. Over time she transformed from a submissive, yielding wallflower to a fiery, outspoken, highly assertive woman with a hilarious sense of humor. Her headaches became a thing of the past.

Agrimony, an astringent belonging to the rose family, is specific for people who feel a sense of inner torment but hide it behind a seemingly happy façade. It is also a highly protective herb, which was important for this patient as her ex-husband tended to be invasive and difficult to deal with. Astringent herbs can be used to tighten the auric web just as they tighten and strengthen mucous membrane sufaces. Potentilla spp. also known as cinquefoil, is another protective astringent that is closely related to agrimony. The five fingered cinqufoil, which has five leaflets and looks something like a human hand, is considered sacred and protective in Celtic tradition. In my experience, cinquefoil is uplifting and empowering for those who need it, as well as protective.

Case

A 45 year old woman with chronic fatigue and fibromyalgia reported having headaches for as long as she could remember and suffered from head pain 90% of the time. Severe headaches were usually left-sided with throbbing sharp pains "like lightning bolts" shooting from the back of her neck to the front of her head. These headaches were often preceded by an aura of flashing lights.

In addition to constitutional treatment, which included homeopathic Natrum muriaticum, a remedy commonly used for headaches, she was given a tincture of 5 parts feverfew and 3 parts lavender to be taken 15 drops 3 times per day. For acute symptoms she was instructed to use same the dose every 15 minutes to every 2 hours as needed and to do a hot foot bath with cold applications to the head whenever practical.

On her return visit 2 weeks later, she reported that her headaches were still constant, but less severe. She noticed that on the days she took the feverfew 4 - 6 times her pain was less intense. Her energy was slightly better, probably as a result of the homeopathic Natrum muriaticum.

The feverfew and lavender tincture was increased to 30 drops 3 times per day. The result was that her headaches were no longer constant and occurred with less and less frequency. Three months later, she reported that her headaches were down to one or two per week and quickly resolved with an extra dose or two of the herbs. On one occasion I shared with her that I had originally been taught to use feverfew only for preventing headaches, as it was not considered effective for treating acute headache symptoms. Her response was passionate. "Well!" she exclaimed, "Those doctors should have talked to the patients who take feverfew!"

Case

A 35 year old woman reported to clinic complaining of frequent headaches and "weird digestion." She stated that she had a tendency to get diarrhea after eating lettuce, spicy or fatty foods, raw broccoli, or onions. She also experienced rumbling in her abdomen followed by diarrhea if she was stressed or anxious.

Headaches occurred once a week and could be quite severe with throbbing pain and a feeling that her "head would explode."

This patient was given a single dose of homeopathic Lycopodium 200 C and a tincture of 4 parts feverfew, 3 parts lavender and one part ginger, to be taken with meals, 30 drops, 2 times per day.

Another formula which included 2 parts Avena sativa, 2 parts Eleutherococcus senticosis, and 4 parts of Silybum marianum was also dispensed. The Eleutherococcus and Avena were given to support her adrenal function as she was under a fair amount of stress. In addition, the Avena was chosen for its actions as a nutritive nervine while the Silybum was given as a restorative healing plant for the liver, as chronic intestinal symptoms generally contribute to liver congestion.

On her follow up visit 4 weeks later she reported that her intestinal symptoms were better almost immediately after taking the Lycopodium, and she had only had two headaches since her first office call, both of which were quickly resolved by a 30 drop dose of the feverfew formula, which she repeated one hour later, when symptoms threatened to return.

Over the next few months this patient was able to eat all the foods she had formerly been unable to assimilate. The digestive stimulating properties of the feverfew and lavender combined well with ginger's carminative actions and the ability of the homeopathic Lycopodium to stimulate healing of the digestive tract.

Petasites spp. (Butterbur, Western Coltsfoot) Asteraceae

Another herb useful for toxic or migraine headaches is Petasites. The leaves, roots, and rhizomes are used, and contain various constituents including mucilage, saponins, two sesquiterpenes (petasin and isopetasin), flavonoids, tannins, resins, essential oils, and bitters. Pyrrolizidine alkaloids may be present in young leaves with little to none found in more mature leaves.[92] Because these particular alkaloids have been associated with severe veno-occlusive liver disease in some individuals, it is probably safest to use a pyrrolizidine free extract.

Petasites prefers moist shady forests. Its large palmate leaves shade out any potential undergrowth, although the occasional brave Equisetum will sometimes be seen popping up here and there in a stand of Petasites. The name Petasites translates from Greek to refer to a large broad brimmed hat commonly worn by shepherds.

Most of the research has been done on P. hybridus, although other species of the plant have been used successfully for all the same indications. Other species include P. palmatus, P. sagittatus, P. frigidies, and P. vulgaris.

Historically, the most common use of Petasites spp. has been for the treatment of spasmodic coughs, as is seen with asthma, chronic obstructive pulmonary disease (COPD), pertussis (whooping cough), and bronchitis. The sesquiterpene petasin is credited with giving the plant its spasmolytic activity. Petasin has also been shown to inhibit leukotriene and lipoxygenase pathways, making it useful in alleviating excessive inflammation. Isopetasin, another sesquiterpene present in Petasites, is also active in prostaglandin pathways to modulate inflammation. [93,94]

Studies have shown significant improvement in lung ventilation as evidence by pulmonary function tests in chronic obstructive pulmonary disease (COPD) and asthma. The plant has also been shown to be effective in the treatment of seasonal allergic rhinitis, (hay fever) where we may presume that the combined effects of flavonoids and sesquiterpenes give the plant anti-inflammatory and anti-allergic actions.[95]

Petasites has long been used as an anti-spasmodic in the urinary tract, biliary tree, gastrointestinal tract, respiratory tract, and uterus. Although I have not uncovered any references to the use of Petasites in the treatment of hypertension, there is some suggestion that the plant's spasmolytic activity may extend to the vasculature as well.

Petasites has been used to treat and help prevent gastric and duodenal inflammation. Weiss suggests that the plant may be dosed by the tablespoonful for "gastrocardiac syndrome," an old term used to refer to gastroesophageal reflux. Because overloaded detoxification pathways render many modern patients less able to process pyrrolizidine alkaloids, such heroic dosing might not be advisable any more unless PA free extracts are utilized.

As an analgesic, Petasites has been employed to relieve lumbosacral and intercostal pain, and pain associated with herniated disc, cervical thoracic outlet syndrome, migraines, and end stage cancer.

Petasites is currently being used to reduce incidence, severity, duration, and frequency of migraine. Some sources suggest an affinity for cerebral blood vessels where the plant's spasmolytic and anti-inflammatory properties prevent and relieve symptoms of migraine. Experience in clinic has revealed Petasites to be helpful in preventing and treating headaches that occur as a result of biliary stasis. Pain in the trapezius muscles of the upper back and shoulder may radiate upward along the path of the gall bladder meridian, causing headache. Nausea and vomiting are not infrequent in these cases.

Michael Moore reports that topical use of Petasites results in anti-inflammatory, antiseptic, and analgesic actions when used as a vulnerary. It may also inhibit bruising and edema of tissues at the site of injury.

Maud Grieve in her two volume work "A Modern Herbal," tells us that the seeds of Petasites are reputed to have been used in weaving a spell to attract love into one's life. She does warn that such a ritual is a "bold, desperate, and presumptuous undertaking!" with which I heartily agree. Love should, above all, be a free-choice sort of affair.

Dosage of a 1:2 tincture of fresh herb can be given at 30 - 60 drops as often as 5 times per day to allay symptoms of spasm. Doses of 5 - 30 drops three times per day are often sufficient for prevention of migraine, congestive headache, or biliary stasis.

Fifty to a hundred milligrams taken twice daily for 4 - 6 months of an extract standardized to contain 15% petasin has been recommended for migraine prevention, although I have found the simple tincture to be quite effective.

This plant should not be used in patients with compromised liver function as even the small amount of pyrrolizidine alkaloids present in the plant may be too much for many people, particularly if phase II liver detoxification pathways are compromised. Although most of the studies suggest that levels of pyrrolizidine alkaloids do not appear to be high in this plant a pyrrolizidine-free extract is probably a much safer way to take this plant in these toxic, liver-challenging times. Unless a pyrrolizidine-free preparation is available, Petasites should only be used for a few days in low doses, if at all. The constituent petasin has also been associated with hepatotoxicity but only at doses far above anything normal (200 times the normal dose in one study).[96]

Menorrhagia

In the treatment of menorrhagia, it is important to identify and treat underlying etiologies such as fibroid tumors of the uterus, adenomyosis, endometriosis, pelvic inflammatory disease, estrogen and progesterone imbalances, and low thyroid function. Menopause may produce flooding with menses if either liver stagnation and/or adrenal fatigue are contributing to create estrogen dominance and actual or relative progesterone deficiency. Reproductive cancers can also present as menorrhagia, and although they are not as common as less life-threatening conditions, they are certainly not rare.

Interestingly, iron deficiency can be an etiologic factor in menorrhagia, in which case, supplementing iron will resolve symptoms of excessive bleeding. The use of anti-biotics may destroy intestinal flora necessary to synthesize vitamin K, a nutrient essential for clotting. Supplemental vitamin K and oral probiotic therapy may be indicated to correct resultant menorrhagia in these women. It is also important to rule out the excessive use of aspirin or anticoagulant drugs as the cause of a woman's excessively heavy menses.

The diagnosis of hormone imbalance should be made only as being secondary to another cause, either lesional or functional. It has been my experience that the use of exogenous hormone therapy to treat these women is simply treating a symptom without addressing the underlying cause and is rarely, if ever, necessary when good naturopathic therapies are employed. Liver stagnation, adrenal fatigue, and pelvic congestion may all contribute to hormonal imbalances or lesions that result in menorrhagia.

Treatment of menorrhagia includes improving liver and adrenal function as well as addressing uterine symptoms. Pelvic decongestant formulas should empahsize styptic herbs such as Achillea, Ceanothus, Alchemilla and Capsella. Since estrogen dominance and/or progesterone deficiency are often present, progestogenic herbs such as Vitex, Smilax, and Dioscorea should also be considered. Biphasic formulas discussed in the next section may also be helpful.

Perhaps one of our most prominent hormonal modulators in herbal medicine is chaste tree berry (Vitex agnus castus). Vitex works by enabling the pituitary gland to increase LH (luteinizing hormone) ultimately leading to an increased production of progesterone, which may be helpful where excessive or irregular bleeding are present. In menopause Vitex serves by inhibiting FSH (follicle stimulating hormone) where it may be helpful in reducing hot flashes. Vitex is regulatory to the menstrual cycle and may be used in amenorrhea, infertility, excessive bleeding, excessively long or short cycles, PMS, and fibroids.

Angelica sinensis (dong quai) is contraindicated in women with a tendency to excessively heavy menses and should not be used in cases where menorrhagia is an issue.

Constitutional homeopathy is invaluable in the treatment of menorrhagia. Some of the more common homeopathic remedies that have proven useful in this prescriber's clinical practice include Lycopodium, Phosphorus, Aurum muriaticum natrum and Cimicifuga.

Calcarea carbonica, Phosphorus, and Sepia

Many physicians feel the necessity to resort to hormones to control menstrual hemorrhage while correcting underlying liver stagnation, nutritional and digestive health, and adrenal insufficiency. Certainly a woman cannot be allowed to bleed herself into a significant anemia while underlying constitutional issues are being addressed, but there are highly effective nonhormonal options available to us for modulating excessive bleeding.

In most cases, homeopathic Sabina 200C taken every 4 - 6 hours as needed for excessive bleeding will be highly effective at reducing hemorrhage without suppressing the healing process. It is important to stress to the woman that the remedy is only meant to allay serious bleeding, not stop bleeding altogether. The use of Sabina circumvents the need to prescribe progesterone, a hormone often given to staunch hemorrhagic bleeding during menses.

On a rare occasion, when Sabina does not do the trick, homeopathic Cimicifuga may be indicated for the acute bleeding. Phosphorus is another remedy I have used when constitutional symptoms fit.

A tincture of astringent herbs can be added at doses of 30 - 60 drops every 1 - 2 hours as needed for excessive bleeding. Herbs to consider for inclusion in an astringent formula include Achillea, Geranium, Capsella, Ceanothus, Cinnamonum, Agrimonia, Alchemilla, and Erigeron.

Amenorrhea, Metrorrhagia, and Irregular Cycles

Bleeding between menses (metrorrhagia), irregular cycles, or absence of menses (amenorrhea) are conditions that are most often related to hormonal imbalances, liver congestion, adrenal fatigue, and/or thyroid imbalances. As always, it is important that underlying pathologies are ruled out before assuming that the problem is simply a question of re-establishing proper organ function.

There are two types of amenorrhea. Primary amenorrhea is a condition where there has been no menses by the age of 16. Before the age of 16, irregularity in menses is normal as the body transitions through adolescence into womanhood. Primary amenorrhea is fairly uncommon and can be due to genetic or structural problems, or from dysfunction in the hypothalamus or pituitary glands. The latter can be due to a tumor or simply as a result of extreme over-exercise, high stress, or an eating disorder.

Secondary amenorrhea refers to cases where there is a cessation of menses after a woman has previously had periods. This type of amenorrhea is more common than primary amenorrhea and is usually not due to serious disease.

Pregnancy, lactation, and menopause are normal causes of amenorrhea. Lactation will normally delay the return of menses after childbirth. Abnormal causes of secondary amenorrhea include, but are not limited to, excessive stress, low thyroid function, poly cystic ovarian syndrome (PCOS), ovarian failure (often erroneously called "early menopause"), habitual over-exercise, eating disorders, and low body weight. Hormonal birth control and some medications can also suppress menstrual flow.

Irregular cycling or bleeding between menses can be due to a variety of things including stress, low thyroid function, over-exercise, significant changes in weight, high carbohydrate diets, liver congestion, various pharmaceutical medications, eating disorders, polycystic ovarian syndrome, and sometimes uterine disorders such as fibroids, polyps, or endometriosis. Irregular cycling is normal during adolescence, lactation, and perimenopause. The occasional missed period in a normally menstruating woman is not generally cause for alarm.

Biphasic Formulas for Menorrhagia and Irregular Menses

In addition to addressing underlying causes, hormonal balancing can be achieved by the use of biphasic formulas. With this approach, a woman may take a formula of herbs that supports estrogen production for the first two weeks of the cycle, followed by a second formula of progesterogenic herbs for the last two weeks. These herbs do not act like hormones in the body. Instead they feed the hormonal pathways and tonify related organs so the body has what is needed to synthesize the appropriate hormones and restore normal function.

Formula I in a biphasic protocol is started on day one of the cycle (the first day of menses). For a woman with amenorrhea, the first formula should be started with the new moon.

Formula I might consist of herbs such as:

Actea (Cimicifuga) racemosa (Black Cohosh)
Medicago sativa (Alfalfa)
Angelica sinensis (Dong Quai)
Foeniculinum vulgare (Fennel Seed).

Days 1-15 (or at new moon) the formula is taken 30-60 drops 3 times per day then discontinued for the next two weeks.

Formula II is started on day 16 (or the full moon) and continued through day 28 of the cycle. The herbs in this formula might include:

Disocorea villosa (wild yam)
Vitex agnus-castus
Smilax spp.
Glycerrhiza glabra
Trigonella foenum-graecum (fenugreek seeds)

This formula is also dosed at 30 - 60 drops three times per day for two weeks, after which the patient returns to Formula I continuing in this fashion until normal cycles are well established and for a time thereafter.

Alternatively, rotation of various seeds and oils has been used with good success in regulating cycles. Seeds are ground fresh in a coffee grinder each day and 2 tablespoons of the ground seeds appropriate for that time of the cycle are used. When measuring seeds it is important to measure the ground seeds, as whole seeds will weigh differently.

Seeds for Phase I of the cycle are flax or pumpkin. Essential fatty acids for this phase are fish oils taken 1 -3 teaspoons daily. (Four capsules of the oil may be considered equal to one teaspoon of the liquid.) Seeds for Phase II of the cycle include sesame or sunflower seeds, while the oils that are used are evening primrose oil (dosage to equal 130 mg. of GLA) and only I teaspoon of the fish oil.

Because Vitex works so well at normalizing hormone imbalances in the female reproductive system, it is actually nice to administer it all month long. When Vitex is included in both formulas, the dose should be doubled in the formula used for the luteal phase. (Formula II). Although I often dose adrenal and liver herbs in separate formulas, a bit of Arctium lappa (burdock root) or Taraxacum officinalis (dandelion root) can be added to both formulas for further hormonal modulation, alterative actions, and liver support. When Glycerrhiza is included in the first formula, the adrenals will be nourished to some degree. Another adaptogen, such as Uncaria tomentosa (cat's claw) could be added to the second formula. I like to see these patients getting at least 30 to 60 drops of adrenal herbs 3 times per day, so I frequently include adrenal herbs in a separate formula.

Seeds must be raw to have effect and when oils are used they should be of good quality and taken with food.

Some physicians use homeopathic nosodes for stimulating a return to normal cycling. As I generally prefer to use a constitutional remedy combined with the biphasic formula of herbs and/or seeds and oils for my patients I have rarely found it necessary to use the following protocol. However I would not hesitate to do so if I was not achieving desired results with my usual approach.

One dose of a 200K of each remedy is taken away from food on the indicated day as listed below.

Hypophysinum 200 K on day one (new moon)
Folliculinum 200 K on day 8
Ovarinum 200 K on day 15 (full moon)
Luteinum 200 K on day 22

This homeopathic protocol will work best if given in conjunction with the biphasic herbal formulas, seeds and/or essential fatty acids.

Bacterial Vaginosis

Bacterial vaginosis is an imbalance of bacteria in the vaginal canal that results in a yellowish, malodorous discharge. The discharge is usually bland, and although the rare woman will report some irritation, in general the discharge is painless

Although this common condition is usually treated as a vaginal infection, it is actually a result of pelvic stagnation and liver sluggishness. Treating the symptoms with strong anti-biotics or herbal douches does not address the underlying etiology and may cause suppression of symptoms rather than cure. Recurrence is frequent with local treatment. The presence of bacteria reflects a condition of dysbiosis that occurs as a result of toxemia and pelvic congestion. Killing off undesirable bacteria does nothing to address the root cause.

A forty two year old woman, who had developed symptoms of bacterial vaginosis, liver tenderness and chemical sensitivity after working for six months in a dry cleaning facility, used a douche of strong anti-septic herbs to rid herself of the discharge. Within a week she experienced a large lump in her breast and her dependably regular and scanty period arrived a week early attended by fairly heavy bleeding. When her body's effort to release toxins though the vaginal discharge was subverted, the process was forced to a deeper level, causing the body to resort to a more pathological discharge (excessive bleeding instead of vaginal symptoms) and create a cyst to deposit toxins. Nature will do her best to discharge toxins in the least harmful way possible, but when we interfere with that process, the body will still attempt to heal through elimination of toxic materials.

A formula of pelvic decongestant herbs taken 30 - 60 drops three to four times per day nearly always clears up the discharge, especially when combined with liver support and the appropriate dietary changes. Pelvic exercises such as yoga, belly dancing, Kegels, and horseback riding should be encouraged. These simple non-toxic therapies work by mobilizing lymph and blood flow thereby moving accumulated toxins out of the pelvis to more appropriate organs of elimination.

In stubborn cases, the insertion of a vitamin A suppository followed by what is known to naturopathic doctors as a vaginal depletion pack or "vag pack," are left overnight in the vaginal canal to pull toxins from the pelvic cavity. This pack, which is made of a combination of mineral salts and essential oils, aids the body in its attempt to discharge toxins, by pulling the toxins out of the pelvis. The discharge is temporarily eliminated as it is no longer necessary to eliminate toxins.

The traditional "vag pack" compound can be purchased by physicians from Eclectic Institute in Sandy, Oregon. It comes as a thick syrupy mixture which is dispensed to the patient with instructions to place approximately a quarter to a half teaspoonful onto the center of a 4" by 4" gauze pad. This is then tied like a hobo bundle with a piece of dental floss. The floss should be tied in such a fashion that one string is left longer to remove the pack in the morning. A vitamin A suppository is inserted high into the vagina before inserting the pack. The vitamin A is important to protect the cervix from the caustic nature of the mineral salts in the pack.

The pack is left in the vagina overnight. Although the herbs in the compound are strong anti-septics, suppression is not an issue since the main action of the pack is to draw toxins from the area. This pack is repeated as needed whenever the discharge returns, perhaps once or twice weekly at most. A pad should be worn overnight with the pack as leakage is common. The pack is pleasant smelling due to the presence of anti-microbial essential oils.

Although there are generally no problems with the pack, the treatment should not be continued if the woman experiences burning in the vagina with the pack. The pack should always be used in conjunction with a formula of pelvic decongestant herbs.

Most cases of bacterial vaginosis will respond to a tincture of pelvic decongestant herbs taken orally and will not require the use of the vaginal depletion pack. Musculoskeletal fixations of the pelvic floor should be corrected as such fixations can prove to be an obstacle to cure. Many physical therapists are trained in intravaginal pelvic floor release. These treatments can be remarkable when indicated.

Candida vaginitis is a different situation altogether and may be treated quite safely with intravaginal therapies, such as boric acid suppositories and probiotics or by inserting a clove of garlic into the vagina overnight. A piece of dental floss should be wrapped around a clove of garlic. The loose end of the floss is left long enough to hang out of the vaginal canal for ease in removing the garlic in the morning. Attention to digestive health, intestinal dysbiosis, and carbohydrate metabolism are integral to successful treatment of recurrent candida vaginitis.

Homeopathic Kreosotum alone, without intravaginal treatment, will often clear up an acute case of candida vaginitis. It will not address the tendency to recurrence however and underlying issues will still need to be corrected. Oral ingestion of probiotics can help tendencies to Candida overgrowth. The homeopathic Kreosotum may be dosed 30C every 2 - 4 hours for 24 hours while awake, followed by every 4 - 6 hours as needed for 24 hours. If the remedy is going to work, positive results should be seen within 24 hours. I have never seen it act suppressively.

Ovarian Cysts and Polycystic Ovarian Syndrome

Any patient with ovarian cysts, polycystic or not, should avoid methylxanthines found in coffee, chocolate, and kolas. These alkaloids will definitely aggravate the condition and create an obstacle to cure in treatment. Methylxanthines are also present in some medications prescribed for asthma.

Because ovarian cysts are generally due to a condition of hyperestogenism, enhancing liver function is essential for clearing excess buildup of hormones. Healthy adrenal cortical function is also essential for optimal hormone balance. A well selected homeopathic remedy will do wonders in clearing pelvic congestion when coupled with liver and adrenal support, as well as a good formula of pelvic decongestant herbs. In treating polycystic ovarian syndrome (PCOS), dietary changes that address food sensitivities and insulin resistance are essential for positive results, as elevated blood glucose and elevated insulin are one of the main contributing factors to the development of PCOS.

Glycerrhiza glabra should be considered for inclusion in adrenal formulas for the treatment of polycystic ovarian syndrome (PCOS) as it has been shown to lower testosterone with long term use and may be of service in modulating elevations in testosterone associated with PCOS. Licorice has also been shown to aid in reducing the side effects of spironolactone, a medication often prescribed for the management of PCOS.[97]

Ceanothus spp. is specific for cysts and should be considered as a primary pelvic decongestant along with Serenoa repens in any woman presenting with polycystic ovarian syndrome.

Serenoa repens, also a pelvic decongestant, is particularly helpful in modulating abnormal testosterone levels that often occur with polycystic ovarian syndrome.

An effective pelvic decongestant formula can be made from 3 - 4 herbs that suit the particular patient and dosed 30 - 60 drops 3 - 4 times per day.

Vitex agnus castus should be considered to enhance progesterone pathways and help regulate hormone balance.

Cinnamon may be included for its positive effects in modulating the insulin resistance that generally accompanies PCOS.

Protocols for amenorrhea and dysmenorrhea, outlined at the beginning of this chapter will prove useful in mitigating symptoms while underlying constitutional work is being done.

Chapter 13
Optimizing Breast Health

BREAST TISSUE IS LARGELY LYMPHATIC IN NATURE, and although many herbs have lymphatic activity, Ceanothus spp. and Viola odorata appear to have more specificity for breast lymphatics than many other herbs.

Symptoms of lymphatic congestion in breasts include cyst formation, fibrocystic breast syndrome, and premenstrual breast tenderness.

Breast tissue does not differ from other organs in its relation to the body as a whole functioning organism. Healthy breast tissue is not independent of gastrointestinal, adrenal, thyroid, liver, or immune function. As always, the needs of the whole individual must be addressed for optimal health to exist.

Located in the area of the heart chakra, breast health is often intimately related to the balance of giving and receiving. Experience in clinic has shown that imbalances in breast health often correlate with giving too much, not listening to the inner voices that recommend saying no instead of yes, or being forced into a situation where we are manipulated into dealing with a draining, sucking energy despite all attempts to say no. Breast health is also related to our ability to be receptive and open ourselves to be vulnerable enough to allow others to give back.

SELF BREAST EXAM

At this writing official recommendations have changed to advise against self breast exam. My clinical experience suggests that this is unwise and even foolish. Self breast exam not only offers women an opportunity to explore and bring love to their bodies, but is the only early detection we have that can be done monthly with no financial cost to the patient. While technology is undoubtedly an invaluable and often essential asset in the diagnosis and early detection of various health conditions, we have, as a culture, become increasingly dependent on technology based methods of assessment, relying less and less on physical touch and our own experience. Self breast exam offers women an opportunity to take a bit of their power back from technology and develop a relationship with their bodies that goes beyond looking for a possible pathology.

Self-breast exam does not need to be a dreaded ritual during which we approach our breasts each month in trepidation and fear of finding early signs of a potentially deadly disease. While scanning for changes is certainly an essential part of the exam, self breast exam also offers us an opportunity to nourish, love, and listen to our bodies regularly. Using herbal oils such as Hypericum, Calendula, Taraxacum, Arctium, Trifolium, Viola, Plantago, or Achillea for gentle lymphatic massage can be beneficial on many levels as we take time to listen and appreciate the beauty of our breasts.

In acknowledgement of the increased openness and sensitivity that occurs during menstruation, European women historically rubbed an infused oil of Hypericum onto the labia during menses for spiritual protection. The red flavonoids that add such rich color to the oil also contribute physically protective properties. Such spiritual protection can surely be applied to our heart/breast chakra as well.

Achillea is protective to highly sensitive and receptive folks who easily feel the wounds of others.

Plantago lanceolata or majus has a reputation for preventing the development of breast cancer when used topically.

Phytolacca spp. should be reserved for application to breast lumps rather than as a general nourishing herb in self-breast exam. A strong herb, it has been known to cause a skin rash in some sensitive people.

Essential Oils in Self Breast Exam

The healing properties of aromatherapy that come through inhalation of plant essential oils cannot be underestimated. The pleasant odor emitted by the aroma of the oils stimulates the olfactory nerve, which in turn feeds directly into the limbic system, a deep emotional center in the brain. The addition of a few drops of essential oil to the herbal oil being used for self breast exam can affect mental, emotional, and spiritual aspects of the patient in subtle but often profound ways.

While Thuja occidentalis (cedar) and Juniperus virginica (juniper) are especially reputed to have anticancer activity, any evergreen essential oil can be beneficial. Other oils like citrus or lavender may also be used. The best oil is the one that suits the patient's olfactory senses. Selection of oils can be varied month to month in accordance with the woman's mood and intuition.

Finally, no matter how good the doctor is, he or she is never as skilled at finding the tiny lump in her breast as a woman who has become familiar with her own body through regular self breast exam. I have seen patients come in with small lumps that were difficult for the physician to find even when the patient was pointing the lump out, and I have been one of those patients myself. While we all need to respect those who have medical experience and have worked hard to gain their skills, it is important that we not give all of the expertise over to practitioners. As a culture we need to remember that technology is not always accurate and, in the case of mammography, not necessarily the safest screening tool. I still recommend that all my patients reclaim their power and knowledge of their own bodies and do a loving breast self-exam monthly.

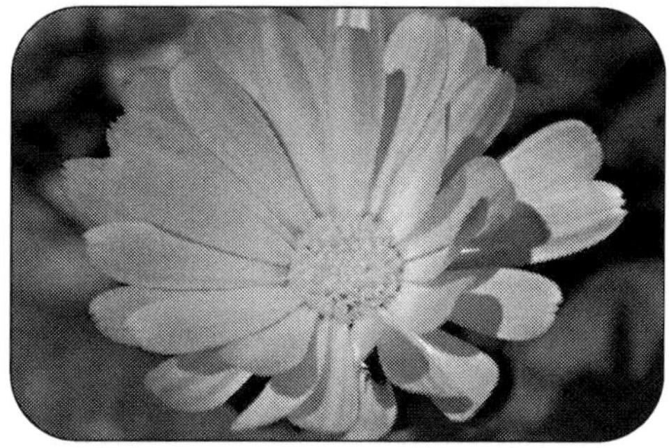

Calendula *Photo courtesy of Orna Izakson N.D.*

Nourishing Herbs for Breast Tissue

Dark green leafy vegetables are masters at bringing light into physical form through the process of photosynthesis. Seaweeds, high in a variety of nutrients including many minerals and iodine are some of the richest dark green leafy vegetables available to us.

One protocol for the treatment of fibrocystic breast syndrome includes supplemental iodine. Seaweeds are a great food source of iodine, a nutrient known to be protective to breast and ovarian tissue as well as vital for proper thyroid function. Selenium, an anti-oxidant deficient in the soils in many areas, is another essential nutrient shown to be protective in the prevention of breast cancer. As excessive selenium can be toxic, doses should be limited to 200 micrograms per day unless otherwise recommended by a qualified health care practitioner.

Ceanothus is my favorite herb for treating premenstrual breast tenderness. It should be taken all month long, to prevent lymphatic stagnation and keep energy moving. Ceanothus is also decongestant in the pelvis, liver, other lymph tissue, and spleen. Flavonoid content helps to protect and strengthen blood vessels, where capillary fragility may be contributing to easy bruising or excessive menstrual bleeding. Dosage of tincture is 15 drops 3 times per day to be taken throughout the month, not just at the time of symptoms. Although higher doses of up to 60 drops three times per day can be implemented, it is rarely necessary and sometimes less efficacious.

The leaves of Viola odorata may also be used with confidence for the treatment of premenstrual breast tenderness. This pretty little plant is an excellent lymphogogue, is anti-viral, and has been used as an expectorant in respiratory illnesses. Its anticancer activity is specific for breast tissue, although it should also be considered for cancers in the gastrointestinal tract where its action as a lymphogogue may be mobilizing lymphatic flow in the rich mesentery surrounding the intestines.

As with Ceanothus, the flavonoid content of Viola lends a protective quality to its healing properties. The leaves are mild tasting and do well when taken as a tea, 1 teaspoon of leaf per cup of water, then drinking 2 cups per day all month long. Although either herb taken alone is generally adequate, they can be combined in stubborn cases. Other constituents of Viola include saponins and glycosides.

Methylxanthines present in coffee, kolas, and chocolate contribute to cystic growths and should be discontinued whenever breast tenderness, ovarian cysts, or uterine fibroids are part of the picture.

Chapter 14

From Mother to Elder: Menopause as Sacred Transition

"Women in the United States report more hot flashes than women from developing countries, where menopause generally seems to be associated with fewer complaints."

Philip, Hazel, N.D., L.Ac, "Hot Flashes A Review of the Literature on Alternative and Complimentary Treatment Approaches," Alternative Medicine Review, Vol. 8, No. 3, August 2003, p. 284

"(Ceremonial) rites were often governed by old women, due to the ancient belief that post¬menopausal women were the wisest of mortals because they permanently retained their wise blood. In the 17th century A.D., Christian writers still insisted that old women were filled with magic power because their menstrual blood remained in their veins. This was the real reason why old women were constantly persecuted for witchcraft. The same magic blood that made them leaders in the ancient clan system made them objects of fear under the new patriarchal faith."

Walker, Barbara, "The Womens Encyclopedia of Myths & Secrets", Book Sales Inc., 1996, p. 641

Throughout the ages traditional cultures have used plants to nourish women through all aspects of our cycles, from puberty, through each menstrual period, certainly in pregnancy, and finally again in menopause.

A few mild hot flashes, night sweats, or a bit of vaginal dryness may just be the body's way of calling out for support during a critical transition. Indeed many women still go through menopause with only a few mild symptoms, but for others, symptoms of hot flashes, emotional lability, insomnia, vaginal dryness, foggy headedness, menorrhagia, (hemorrohagic menstrual bleeding), joint pains, and decreased thyroid function are becoming more common due to the ever increasing pollutants in the environment and a modern world that is out of touch with the normal cycles of the women's bodies and of nature generally.

The only "normal" symptoms of menopause are cessation of menses. All other symptoms are a sign of imbalance. As bleeding cycles ease off and finally cease, women may experience yet another pull to introspection and Earth body awareness that offers tremendous potential for physically incorporating a deeper sense of wisdom and spiritual connection. This powerful process can be enhanced by nourishing our bodies with good food, appropriate herbal medicines, and a healthy lifestyle. As with anything else, the basic principles of a healthy diet, adequate sleep, exercise, fresh air, sunshine, and emotional and spiritual nourishment provide an essential foundation for all other treatments.

The normal age for menopause is somewhere near the age of fifty and unless a woman has a family history of early menopause, cessation of menses before the late forties may be a result of other underlying issues, such as chemotherapy or radiation for cancer treatment, complete hysterectomy, malnutrition, illness, severe stress, or exposure to environmental pollutants.

Nourishing the Transition

Most women who are symptomatic with menopause will benefit from a formula of herbs that nourish and tone the female endocrine system. Angelica sinensis (dong quai), Asparagus racemosa (shatavari), and Medicago sativa (alfalfa) are good, nourishing foundational herbs. Other plants may be included as indicated by symptoms. Adding more legumes to the diet will also help support a healthy transition, as these foods are high in phytoestrogenic constituents that nourish hormonal pathways.

Adrenal, liver, and thyroid support are often key to a successful treatment plan for the symptomatic woman. Ideally, I like to evaluate women a few years before menopause to restore optimal function to endocrine organs ahead of time.

Hot Flashes

Many women have little to no problem with hot flashes while others struggle with uncomfortable surges of heat and night sweats.

One woman managed her hot flashes simply by increasing the legumes in her diet, but for others that may not be enough. Vitamin E in doses of 400 - 800 I.U.s and hisperidin may be of help for some women.

Hot flashes come as surges of power, encouraging us to stand up for ourselves, demand the respect we deserve, and step into new levels of assertiveness. As a symptom, flushes of heat are often associated with the liver. It is no coincidence that this organ is located in the area of the solar plexus, known in Yogic traditions as the 3rd chakra, the center of personal power. For women, there are many, deeply ingrained, subtle and not so subtle, social taboos to taking power. Fortunately, this pattern is changing, as women move into more roles of responsibility and leadership in the world and the Feminine Principle is beginning to resurrect in collective consciousness, demanding respect for all life.

Nourishing and supporting liver function is therefore essential when hot flashes are present. Liver congestion can occur for a variety of reasons. Poor diet, inadequate sleep, lack of exercise, lack of love and self appreciation, and exogenous toxins are a few examples of things that can interfere with optimal liver function. Suppression of an appropriate expression of the inner spirit that demands transcendence of culturally imposed limitations can also cause stagnation in liver Qi. Suppression of our vitality/fire ultimately can also lead to emotional depression.

Black cohosh (Cimicifuga/Actea racemosa) has proven itself to be one of my most reliable remedies for alleviating hot flashes. It works well when combined in a formula with the nourishing herbs mentioned above and taken four times per day, where it also may serve to prevent bone loss.[98] In addition, a separate bottle of Cimicifuga alone can be dispensed with instructions to take 5 - 15 drops as needed for hot flashes. Patients should be instructed to decrease dosing if a dull frontal headache occurs. Tolerance varies with individual needs and may shift for the same patient at different stages of healing. While Cimicifuga can be given to any woman who is experiencing significant hot flashes, remember it as a specific when abuse or deep dark depression occur as concomitant symptoms.

One woman who was struggling with trying to end an abusive relationship experienced intense hot flashes when she entered menopause. A wild, chaotic feeling in her mind and great difficulty in concentrating accompanied her hot flashes, coming and going as intensely and abruptly as the surges of heat and profuse sweating. Her symptoms were specific for Cimicifuga and she daily ingested doses at the top of the therapeutic range without a hint of any headache. She was also given an adrenal formula, a good quality B complex with minerals, 1000 milligrams of Vitamin C four times per day, and homeopathic Pulsatilla. A year later, having successfully ended the marriage and feeling healthier in every respect, just half the dose of Cimicifuga she had taken earlier brought on a dull, frontal headache. She no longer needed the herb in the same quantities.

Conversely, a young student of herbal medicine in her early twenties who was a bright, sunny, optimistic person, decided to take a dose of Cimicifuga as part of her learning experience. One dose of 30 drops and she immediately experienced the dull headache. This happy young woman had no need for this dark underworld plant ally, at least not at this phase of her life.

Cimicifuga can also be useful in the treatment of hypertension, and while I usually use it as a supportive herb in my formulas for high blood pressure, one woman in my practice did well with Cimicifuga alone for her hypertension.

When profuse sweating interferes with sleep and threatens to deplete a woman's strength, Salvia officinalis has shown itself to be invaluable when added to a formula for menopause. Constituents include saponins, phytosterols, essential oils, flavonoids, and minerals, making this plant a highly nourishing ally in the treatment of menopausal hot flashes. The plant is also supportive to the liver and digestion.

It is important to treat each woman as an individual, honoring her symptom presentation and avoiding the tendency to lump every perimenopausal female into a catch-all diagnosis of "hormone imbalance."

Cases

A 53 year old woman who was trying to avoid using exogenous hormone therapies came to clinic complaining of severe intractable hot flashes and persistent insomnia. Her sleep was frequently interrupted by hot flashes, and she also reported feeling generally tense and overwrought. She had been taking a formula of herbs including dong quai, shatavari and black cohosh, but symptoms persisted.

Further questioning revealed the loss of a loved one whom she had nursed through a protracted illness in the year or two preceding menopause. Her last menses had occurred a year and a half before the first office call and 6 months prior to the office visit she had fallen from her horse and landed on her head.

"Do you think I need to go on hormones?" she asked.

"No," I replied. "It sounds to me like your symptoms are more related to the central nervous system than hormones. The head injury may well have affected your pineal and/or pituitary glands, creating significant stress in your endocrine system, thereby causing or contributing to any underlying propensity for hormonal imbalance. I think we should address the cause and I bet your symptoms will quickly resolve."

She was placed on a formula of nervines, including tropho-restorative herbs such as Centella asiatica, Hypericum perforatum and Avena sativa, as her primary therapy. Vitex was added to nourish the pituitary gland and regular orthobionomy sessions were initiated to correct any remaining fixations in the cranium. (Orthobionomy is one of several physical therapy modalities that can help release fixations in the cranium and other musculoskeletal areas). Hawthorne was given to address the underlying etiology of grief and a formula of adrenal herbs was administered to help rebuild her adrenal cortex which had been stressed by the months of caregiving and grief. The patient's previously debilitating hot flashes and insomnia began to respond favorably soon after initiating these therapies.

One patient, who suffered intense insomnia with the onset of menopause, obtained only temporary relief from well prescribed naturopathic therapies. In the end, this woman finally slept consistently when she was able to accept the gift of intuition that she shared with her paternal grandmother, but had denied to herself.

Another patient, who had experienced severe grief and trauma in the year or two preceding menopause, was able to sleep but suffered from intense hot flashes with sweating so profuse they threatened to deplete her electrolytes. Her history included a significant exposure to environmental toxins, making detoxification a vital part of her treatment plant, but in the meantime, Salvia officinalis proved invaluable at alleviating her symptoms and preventing depletion of fluids, electrolytes and general vitality.

Yet another patient's hot flashes and insomnia improved when vitamin B 12 injections were added to her treatment protocol.

After presentating a talk on menopause during which I discussed hot flashes as opportunities to integrate power, one of the participants spoke up, objecting that the irritablility she was experiencing with menopause was simply over the top.

"Can you give me an example?" I queried her.

"Well," she replied. "Just the other night, I asked my 10 year old son to pick up his shoes from the middle of the living room floor. I repeatedly asked him to pick up his shoes but he just ignored me. Suddenly I found myself screaming at him, 'Pick up your shoes NOW!!!' It was terrible! I was screaming!"

"What happened then?" I asked her.

"Well," she responded hesitantly, as if realizing something for the first time. "He picked up his shoes."

"Hmmm," I responded. "That sounds pretty good to me."

Menopausal surges of power may be experienced as irritability and sudden bursts of anger, if we are unable to appropriately integrate the level of empowerment our spirit is calling for. Instead of listening to our feelings, most of us, men and women alike, are conditioned to suppress emotion, especially anger, or if we are encouraged to express it, we are often not given tools to express our anger in a constructive manner. In some cases, listening to, dialogueing with, or journaling our feelings of anger can help lead us to achieve the clarity the anger strives to bring. At other times, as with the woman described, the fire of our anger can enable us to stand up for ourselves appropriately in the moment.

In more enlightened models of horse training, requests are made in phases. Ask gently. If there is no response or the horse resists or is disrespectful, ask again, more firmly this time. If the response is still not appropriate, the request becomes more insistent, with the final fourth phase becoming more of a strong demand. This same pattern can be applied to human interactions.

I recall once riding my gelding, Waku, on the trail with a friend on her mare, Hidaya. Because Waku generally loved being the lead horse, I was puzzled when he would not pass the mare we were riding with. Every time I urged him forward, he would immediately pick up the pace, only to slow down just short of passing her. When I glanced at the mare, I noticed her flick her ear ever so slightly in his direction, using more energy than physical motion to warn him that there would be dire consequences if he did not listen. The mare, displeased with his attempts to pass her, did not start by stretching her neck out to bite or thowing out a back leg to kick my gelding, but she let my horse know in no uncertain circumstances that she was willing to go there if that's what it took. Her first phase request was effective because she was willing to go to the fourth phase and my little gelding knew it.

We can learn a lot about wholeness from the animals in our lives.

Vaginal Dryness

While vaginal dryness once responded well to a simple tincture of Avena sativa (milky oat seed) at dosages of 15 drops 3 times per day, it may not be enough for the modern woman who typically has more adrenal fatigue and liver congestion than was once seen in years past. Avena can be added to an adrenal formula, which should be part of the treatment in any case. Then moisturizing herbal suppositories, or an ointment, can be used intra-vaginally every night for a week or two, after which the applications can be decreased to every other night for a week then every third night and so on until the patient discovers the minimum amount of repetitions necessary to keep tissue moist and healthy. It is important to stress that these herbs do their best work when used regularly to keep tissues healthy. Using the ointment or suppositories only as needed for sexual intercourse will not work as well.

The suppository I use most commonly in my clinic is available from Earth's Botanical Harvest at Eclectic Institute in Sandy, Oregon and contains Vitamin E, Cimicifuga, and Dioscorea. Women have also used Stellaria media (chickweed), Vitex, Althea, Smilax, and Glycerrhiza in homemade salves with good effects.

One single woman, in her mid to late fifties who was no longer sexually active, had such intense vaginal dryness and atrophy that the speculum could absolutely not be placed for her bi-annual pap smear. I sent her home with the suppositories, telling her to use them every single night for a month, before returning to clinic for another try. The result was remarkable. Her vaginal tissue was moist and healthy, allowing the examination to be performed without the slightest discomfort.

It is important to keep vaginal tissues healthy to prevent infection and dysbiosis even if women are not sexually active. Vaginal mucosa often reflects the health of bladder mucosa. Dry mucous membranes in the urinary bladder are likely to increase vulnerability to urinary tract infections.

Liver Health

Hot flashes and night sweats are often the body's way of creating an avenue for toxins to be eliminated. In these cases, diaphoresis, or excessive sweating occurs to compensate for a liver that is too overburdened to process the surges of estrogen released during menopause. There are many liver cleansing protocols that include a cleansing diet, regular sweating, colon therapy, and sometimes various powdered nutritional blends that provide protein and nutrients necessary to feed detoxification pathways. Enhancing detoxification corrects the underlying hepatic insufficiency that prevents the liver from properly breaking down hormones, whereas the use of hormone replacement therapy to relieve hot flashes only increases the hormonal burden that the liver must contend with. In the early days of my practice, liver herbs were all that were needed to correct hot flashes. Now that we live in a much more toxic environment, other therapies, such as Cimicifuga, Angelica sinensis, and Salvia officinalis are often needed in addition to restoring optimal liver function.

Equal parts of dandelion (Taraxacum offinalis) and milk thistle seed (Silybum marianum) taken 15 - 30 drops three times daily with meals is often a good place to start a liver cleanse, especially if patients are sensitive or carrying a heavy load of toxins. Alternatively, a stronger formula that includes Chelidonium, Chionanthus, Burpleurum, and/ or Schisandra with the dandelion and milk thistle may be given 15 - 30 drops two to three times daily with meals. Liver stimulating herbs such dandelion, greater celandine, fringe tree and others, should be avoided at bedtime as they may interfere with sleep. Increased liver activity from the herbs can result in a temporary rise of toxins in the bloodstream, which in turn can irritate the nervous system. This release of processed toxins back into the bloodstream facilitates their transport to organs of elimination such as the urinary tract, colon, or sweat glands. Bitter, liver stimulating herbs are best taken with meals, since they enhance digestion as well as stimulate optimal liver function.

Although most of the bitter herbs will enhance gall bladder and digestive function to some degree, Chelidonium is specific for gall bladder stagnation.

Bupleurum and Schisandra add adaptogenic qualities and Schisandra is rich in anthocyanin, providing anti-inflammatory and anti-oxidant activity.

These days, many of us encounter patients who are not strong enough to tolerate stimulating liver herbs, such as Chelidonium, Chionanthus, and even Taraxacum, Bupleurum or Shisandra. In these patients, Silybum marianium, (1 to 3 tablespoons per day of seed ground in blender or coffee grinder), and Curcuma longa, (1/2 tsp powder 2 times a day) may be given for their hepato-protective and antioxidant effects.

Perhaps one of the most important plants for treating the liver is the simple garden beet. Beets contain numerous flavonoids, including catechins, which have been shown to be hepatoprotective. This simple vegetable also helps drain the liver by enhancing gall bladder function and promoting bowel regularity. Both root and leaf can be used in the diet.[99]

Dark green leafy vegetables in the diet, abundant fresh fruits and vegetables of all sorts, blueberries, blackberries, pomegranates, nettles, red clover, spirulina, burdock, seaweeds and other plants can help bind toxins in the blood stream, further lightening the load on the liver.

For the more vital patient, a liver formula with or without lipotropic factors may be all she needs to bring relief for hot flashes.

Chapter 15
Thyroid Function

A WIDE ARRAY OF ENVIRONMENTAL TOXINS and radiation are wrecking havoc with thyroid function. The endocrine shifts that accompany menopause can stress a marginally functioning thyroid, especially if adrenal and liver function are suboptimal. While consideration of thyroid health during menopause did not generally even come up on the radar 15 to 20 years ago, an environment swimming with endocrine and thyroid disrupting chemicals and radiation make thyroid support a must for many women during menopause. The release of thyro-toxic readiation from the meltdown of the nuclear plant in Chernobyl in April of 1986, and the recent nuclear breakdown in Japan (March 2011), make attention to thyroid health a priority for all of us.

Supplementation with seaweeds in the diet or with a few capsules of good quality Fucus spp. (bladderwrack) will provide iodine and trace minerals necessary to nourish the thyroid and keep it healthy. Iodine supplementation is highly controversial, with some writers claiming large doses are essential and quite safe, while others report toxicity. Certainly iodine can be thyrotoxic in large doses and in certain sensitive individuals. Supplying moderate amounts as whole food is probably the safest way to dose this nutrient, although many people do well with potassium iodide in doses of 12 mcg per day.

As with any herb, sources are vital. Heavy metals, and now increased levels of radioactive materials, pose a concern for many health minded individuals, and rightfully so. In addition, commercial seaweeds may be processed with additives or preservatives that do not necessarily make their way into labeling. Trustworthy herb companies and small local gatherers who know their region are best. Two quality sources I have found to be reliable include a small family owned business called Nature Spirit Herbs located in Williams, Oregon, (www.naturespiritherbs.com) and Ryan Drum PhD., educator and seaweed specialist. (www.ryandrum.com)

Remember that song? "the hip bone's connected to the thigh bone…" If a healthy thyroid gland is not supported by optimal liver function and healthy bacterial flora in the intestinal tract, then inactive thyroid hormone (T4) will not be adequately converted to the more active form (T3). In addition gluten sensitivity can initiate an auto-immune attack on the thyroid as the structure of gluten is fairly similar to thyroid tissue.[100] Issues of insulin resistance, when present, must also be addressed. Finally non-hormonal treatment of hypothyroidism can never be successful without supporting adrenal function.

Ashwaghanda (Withania somnifera) is specific for treating low thyroid function, as it has been shown in studies to increase thyroid hormone production. (For more on Ashwaghanda, see the chapter on adrenal adaptogens.)

What follows is a simple protocol that is often successful for the treatment of uncomplicated hypothyroidism, when combined with a constitutional approach.

Hypothyroid Formula

Fucus spp. (Bladderwrack) 3 drams and/or
Nereocystis spp. (Kelp) 3 drams of one or 1.5 drams of each
Arctium lappa (Burdock root) 2 drams
Withania somnifera (Ashwaghanda) 3 drams
Thyroidinum 3X or 6X (homeopathic)
    - 1 pellet placed into any size dispensing bottle
Iris versicolor (Blue Flag)
    - 30 drops per ounce if thyromegaly is present
    - DOSE: 1/2 to 1 teaspoon 3 times per day

Although most species of seaweed can be relied upon to provide a supply of nutrients to enhance thyroid function, two species in particular have been identified as being particularly helpful in enhancing thyroid function. Fucus spp., used in the formula above, contains di-iodotyrosine (DIT) which is essential for production of thyroid hormone, making this seaweed ideal for the treatment of hypothyroidism. Normally the body must convert monoiodotyrosine (MIT) into DIT for use by the thyroid. MIT is found naturally in the amino acid tyrosine.

The Arctium in the formula is added as an alterative, to balance hormone and liver functions.

Withania supports liver and adrenal function and increases thyroid gland production of T4 and possibly T3.[101,102]

The addition of homeopathic thyroidinum activates the formula and enables the treatment to work effectively when the herbs alone do not succeed. This is always added when hypothyroidism is evident. I do not add the homeopathic thyroidinum if I am simply supporting thyroid function in an otherwise euthyroid (normal thyroid) individual who I suspect may need some preventive treatment. These latter cases will probably do well at 1/2 to 1 teaspoon of the formula 2 - 3 times daily, without the Iris versicolor or thyroidinum.

Patients with autoimmune thyroid disease, such as is seen with Hashimoto's thyroiditis, can benefit from this formula as long as blood serum levels of TSH, FT4, and FT3 are not significantly out of range and avoidance of gluten is strictly adhered to.

The formula usually needs to be continued long term in hypothyroid patients and generally I have found that the dose should not be decreased until thyroid markers have been normal for a full year. I then begin by discontinuing the homeopathic thyroidinum first, retesting after 3 months, (sooner if the patient becomes symptomatic) and eventually reducing the formula to 1/2 teaspoon 2 - 3 times per day or simply having the patient continue the Fucus in capsules or tincture at a lower dose. Most patients will need occasional thyroid support throughout their lives, but may not need to continue it on an ongoing basis.

Iris versicolor (Iris, Blue Flag) Liliaceae

The roots and rhizomes of Iris versicolor, native to North American wetlands have potential toxicity, making attention to dosage vital with this herb. Tilgner recommnends 1 - 5 drops of a 1:2 tincture up to 3 times daily and I typically use the upper end of this dosing.

Traditional stories associated with medicinal plants are a common and important part of the herbal practices in Indigenous culture. These stories and beliefs, if we can be humble enough to listen to them, inform us that the Medicine of our plants is much larger than the cerebral "facts and figures information" that we have grown to revere in the modern world.

Iris, the Greek Goddess of Communication, also known as the Rainbow Goddess, facilitates the transfer of messages from the Lower and Under Worlds (which may be psychologically interpreted as various levels of the unconscious) to the Upper Worlds of consciousness. The plant Iris versicolor, often overlooked and underutilized in herbal medicine is very specific and highly effective in reducing thyromegaly (simple goiter or uncomplicated enlargement of the thyroid gland). The plant's connection to a Goddess who facilitates communication from the depths of the unconscious to the conscious mind combines with the not coincidental location of the thyroid gland in the area of the throat chakra, traditionally associated with communication.

This synchronicity is further amplified by a remark made by the late and most revered Dr. John Bastyr N.D. (1912 - 1995), who remarked during a lecture at Bastyr College of Naturopathic Medicine in 1985, that hypothyroidism is common among women because there is so much resistance to the voice of women in patriarchal society. He suggested that women practice speaking against cultural resistance by "singing into the wind."

Due to increased exposure to toxins and radiation in our environment, the incidence of hypothyroidism has increased astronomically in the past few years. The meltdown of a nuclear power plant in Russia (Chernobyl) in 1986 has increased thyroid pathology substantially. The recent nuclear incident in Japan that occurred as a result of the earthquake and subsequent tsunami of 2011 has certainly not helped matters. The incubation period for radiation to affect thyroid function and produce thyroid cancer is roughly twenty years.[103] Nineteen years after the Chernobyl event, many of us noticed that thyromegaly and hypothyroidism, which had been steadily and gradually increasing in incidence, suddenly shot up dramatically. In my own practice, I began to see thyroid cysts and adenomas that I had not ever seen in previous years.

Patriarchal, aristocratic, hierarchical thinking has dominated the world for centuries, wiping out earth-centered cultures and subjugating the earth, plants, animals, women and working class folks to serve this "higher" authority. (Kings, presidents, corporations…) Prophecies from traditional cultures around the world promise a return of the Feminine Principle, not to then lord over the Masculine, but to stand in equality next to him. With the return of the Feminine, the Masculine Principle will also be redeemed and released from the bondage of patriarchal/dominator models. The voices of women, the calling of our heartfelt, deepest feelings, and the wisdom of Indigenous Teachings are all beginning to be heard again as the world moves into the very times that prophecies have foretold. That having been said, the resistance is still strong within each of us as individuals, within family units, communities, and in our nations and planet as a whole. Welcome, Iris versicolor!

Like the pond lilies, which are related to the eastern lotus, Iris often prefers wet boggy areas, shooting up her beautiful blooms from mucky ponds and wetlands, but only after a period of hibernation. Like the Goddess she is named for, Iris teaches us to value the dark murky "lower world" aspects of human experience and to trust the processes that pull us into inner worlds. Hidden in the depths, we may find lost parts of the human soul, longing to sprout and bloom back into consciousness. But while the lotus grows in the middle of the pond, its roots gathering nourishment from the muckiest depths, Iris prefers the edge of the pond or damp areas of the forest, seemingly not needing to dive as deeply into the center of the murkiness. Once out of the underworld, the peaceful pond lily or lotus is content to rest quietly in blissful enlightenment on the surface of the pond, radiating the peace and wisdom it has gathered from the depths to all who might need it. Iris, on the other hand, shoots her blossoms skyward, encouraging active communication from the depths.

Iris also brings protection to the underworld traveler. Matthew Wood, in his book Seven Herbs, Plants as Teachers, tells us the plant can be likened to the iris of the eye, dilating to allow entrance to the depths and contracting again to prevent an overload of negativity from gaining entrance to the soul.

Iris versicolor is an invaluable alterative in the treatment of thyromegaly where thyroid swelling is soft and uncomplicated by adenomatous, cancerous, or cystic lesions. In these cases it should be accompanied by other herbs as indicated for the condition: Fucus and kelp for hypo or euthyroid conditions and Lycopus, Melissa, and Leonurus for hyperthyroidism. I have never seen Iris fail to reduce simple thyromegaly when there are no adenomas , cysts or other complications.

As an alterative, Iris is specifically indicated for liver congestion with inflammation. Its reputed success in the treatment of reactive hypoglycemia may be due to an alterative effect in the liver that allows glycogen to be synthesized adequately in response to changing blood glucose levels.

Like Ceanothus spp., Iris is also specific for splenic congestion, and also like Ceanothus, it is an excellent lymphatic, especially well suited for soft swelling of lymph nodes.

Iris has also been used as a blood cleanser and may be indicated for the treatment of patients with a tendency to infection, or those who suffer with ongoing low-grade, septic conditions. In this respect, Iris is similar to, yet differs from, Baptisia, the latter being useful for both chronic and acute sepsis, while the use of Iris in these conditions has been for more chronic cases.

Some of the old writers report the successful use of Iris in the treatment of acute pancreatitis, especially when accompanied by a burning sensation in the pancreas. In accoradance with the homeopathic principle of Similia Similibus Curantur, like cures like, we find that toxic doses of this plant can cause significant burning anywhere in the digestive tract, while low doses may be used to treat the same symptoms with success. Excessive salivation may also be an indication that Iris can be of help.

Iris stimulates the flow of bile from the gall bladder and may help increase appetite by stimulating digestive function.

Toxic or sick digestive headaches, as well as migraines, may be helped by Iris versicolor. Often there is a sensation of a heavy weight at the back of the neck. The headache is generally in the frontal area, may be preceeded by an aura of blurring in the eyes, and is generally better from slow movement and worse from rest. A concomitant low-grade depression often accompanies the headache. I have used both drop doses of the herb and homeopathic potencies with success in these cases.

Matthew Wood suggests that patients who respond to Iris are usually highly responsible women who are prone to become overwhelmed and depressed as a result of the burdens they carry, hence the sensation of a weight at the back of the neck. My clinical experience confirms this observation and I often find Iris comes up as a good herb in these cases.

Although this plant is very safe, she is dose sensitive. Like the Goddess she is named for and the women who are reclaiming the power of the spoken word, she should be treated and dosed with respect.

Toxic symptoms include nausea and vomiting (the first symptoms of toxicity in most of the dose sensitive plants), burning in any area of the gastro-intestinal tract, diarrhea, and ultimately death.

Chapter 16

Healing Erectile Dysfunction

SINCE THE FEMINIST MOVEMENT took hold in the 1960's and 1970's, there has been much talk about women, women's rights, women's wounds, women's health, women's power, but little attention has been paid to the needs of our male counterpart. In fact, until recently, speaking of men as being wounded was likely to be greeted with derision. Men were the oppressor and women their unwilling victims in a patriarchal society. Such one-sided thinking has only served to deepen the wounds of both men and women, but fortunately for us all, this kind of prejudicial thinking is shifting.

Loss of tribal elder guidance and initiation ceremonies has injured males as surely as it has women. With adolescence, boys experience significant shifts, mentally, spiritually, emotionally and physically. Our cultural lack of understanding of the sacredness of this transition into manhood, combined with our tendency to denigrate the process by joking about "raging hormones", prevents adolescents of both genders from being honored during this time. Such lack of respect reflects our loss of appreciation of the sacred, life-giving, power that is birthed into both males and females during their transition from childhood to adulthood. Loss of appropriate ceremonies, peer companionship, and the guidance of wise elders leaves all too many young men floundering in the face of the sacred warrior/protector archetype that is emerging from within.

There are more and more men writing about the needs of men and boys. Michael Gurian, a clinical psychologist who writes and lectures on the needs of men and boys, describes the issues well in his books, "*Fine Young Men and The Wonder of Boys*". I highly recommend Gurien's work for my male patients, as well as anyone who is in relationship with a man, whether that man is brother, father, son, or the guy down the street. Practitioners who see men, boys, or women in relationship with males in clinical practice will benefit from Gurien's work, as his writing enables us all to deepen our understanding of male identity, the sacred transition into manhood, and the damage the lack of initiation ritual does to men.

Sexual Dysfunction in Men

Underlying causes and contributing factors to the development of erectile dysfunction must always be taken into consideration. Possible cardiovascular causes include hypertension, hyperlipidemia, and atherosclerosis. The risk of developing erectile dysfunction is increased in patients with diabetes, where long-standing hyperglycemia (high blood sugar) leads to damaged innervation and circulation to the penis. The related carbohydrate intolerance of metabolic syndrome and insulin resistance can also increase risk of erectile dysfunction. Regular exercise and appropriate dietary interventions reduce risk in both diabetes and metabolic syndrome.

Erectile dysfunction can also occur as a complication of renal failure, spinal cord injuries, multiple sclerosis, cerebrovascular accidents (stroke), Alzheimer's disease, and possibly Meniere's syndrome. Surgery, radiation or hormonal therapies used in the treatment of pelvic cancers, such as prostate, bladder, or colon cancer can damage pelvic vasculature and organs, which in turn, can manifest as erectile dysfunction. While function may return spontaneously 6 - 18 months after pelvic surgery, naturopathic therapies can promote more rapid healing of tissues, with earlier recuperation and restoration of sexual function.

Hormonal causes of erectile dysfunction include imbalances in prolactin, hypothyroidism, low testosterone levels, low adrenal function, and tumors of the pituitary gland. Renal and hepatic disease can be the underlying etiology of hormonal imbalances, with liver congestion in the absence of frank pathology being another common etiology.

Finally, an evaluation of potential side effects of any pharmaceutical drugs that the patient is taking may reveal an external etiology for erectile dysfunction.

Most patients respond well to a formula of adrenal adaptogens, herbs specific for the treatment of erectile dysfunction, and a constitutional homeopathic remedy. Acupuncture may be used as an alternative or adjunct to homeopathy. Frequently indicated remedies include, but are not limited to, Lycopodium and Sulphur, with Lycopodium being the most common in my experience.

Adaptogenic Herbs Specific for Erectile Dysfunction

Small but clinically significant amounts of sex hormones are secreted by the adrenal cortex, making a healthy adrenal cortex critical for restoring and maintaining normal hormone balance. Some specific adaptogens, including Maca, Ashwaganda, and Ginseng, share a traditional reputation for being powerfully effective as sexually rejuvenating herbs.

For a more in-depth discussion of this group of herbs please refer to the chapter on adrenal adaptogens. A tincture of one or more adaptogens should be dosed at 30 to 60 drops 3 times per day.

Maca (Lepidium meyenii) Brassicaceae

The roots of maca, a nutritious member of the cabbage family, were prized by both European immigrants and indigenous Peruvians for their ability to increase strength, endurance, and sexual function.[104] Maca has a strong reputation for resurrecting waning erectile function. Constituents include iodine and other minerals, tannins, alkaloids, and saponins.

Ashwaghanda (Withania somnifera) Solanaceae

Ashwaghanda is said to bestow the power and vitality of a horse (Ladd). One may presume such a claim refers to a stallion in his prime. It is another one of the adaptogens that is considered more specific for erectile dysfunction in males.

Ashwaghanda is calming to the central nervous system as well as restorative to adreno-cortical and thyroid function.

Ginseng (Panax ginseng) & American Ginseng (Panax quinquefolius) Araliaceae

The ginsengs are specifically indicated for elders. Although the Panax species have some specificity for erectile dysfunction, high popularity of both Asian and North American species has led to overharvesting on both continents. In addition, ginseng can be overstimulating to the nervous system. Alhough these herbs are invaluable when properly prescribed, it is best to use the ginsengs with discretion.

Siberian Ginseng (Eleutherococcus senticosus) Araliaceae

Eleutherococcus has shown itself in clinic to be a solid, reliable ally in enhancing physiological responses to stress. Unlike its relatives in the Panax genus, (Oriental and American ginsengs) Eleutherococcus does not over stimulate the nervous system. Although not generally listed as one of the "sexy" adaptogens, I had one case where it was quite remarkable.

Licorice Root (Glycerrhiza glabra) Fabaceae

Although licorice is an excellent adrenal adaptogen, it should be noted that it may lower testosterone and is therefore contraindicated in men with erectile dysfunction.

Herbs to Enhance Sexual Function

One herbal formula that has worked well in clinic draws on plants from the lush, fertile, jungles of the Amazon. Two of the herbs in the formular, Catuaba and Muira puama, are available at Amazon herb supplieres. All of these herbs can also be used for women struggling with difficulties in achieving orgasm or low libido unresponsive to adaptogens alone.

Ptychopetalum olacoides (Potency Wood or Muira puama) 10 ml
Erythroxylum catuaba (Catuaba) ....10 ml
Turnera aphrodesiatica (Daimiana) ....5 ml
Smilax officinalis (Sarsaparilla) ....5 ml

This formula may be dosed at 30 to 60 drops 2 - 3 times per day and works best when combined with 1 or 2 of the above mentioned adrenal adaptogens also dosed at 60 drops 3 times daily. While some patients may find that this is all that is needed, many will benefit from overall constitutional treatment with vitality enhancing therapies such as accupuncture or homeopathy.

The above herbs combine well to nourish sexual energy and while they often help to improve low libido as well as heal erectile dysfunction, they are not likely to over stimulate or cause an abnormally high increase in sexual desire.

The formula appears to clear pelvic congestion and enhance prostate function. I have also seen symptoms of benign prostatic hypertrophy (BPH) improve significantly with this formula when other naturopathic protocols were not effective.

Ptychopetalum olacoides (Potency Wood or Muira puama)

"Muira puama has a long history in herbal medicine as an aphrodesiac, a tonic for the nervous system, and an antirheumatic and for gastrointestinal disorders."

Taylor, Leslie, Herbal Secrets of the Rain Forest, Prima Health, 1998, p. 161

A neuroprotective nerve tonic, potency wood has been shown to decrease oxidative damage to brain cells, increasing cognition and memory.[105] It also has anti-depressant actions, at least in part through these same mechanisms.[106] A study done in France in the 1990s tested 262 men with low libido or inability to obtain or maintain an erection. 62% of the men with low libido reported very significant increase in desire, while 51% with actual erectile difficulties reported that the herb was beneficial.[107] Potency wood has a traditional history of use for erectile dysfunction and has certainly proven valuable in clinic. There is probably also some adaptogenic activity involved with the plant, although it seems to be most effective when combined with other adaptogens.

For women the plant has proven useful for menstrual disturbances, symptoms of PMS, infertility, menstrual cramping, and lowered libido.

Constituents include sterols, alkaloids, free fatty acids, essential oil, terpenes, gums, resins. Toxicity is low. (Taylor)

Epimedium spp. (Horny Goat's Weed) Yin Yang Huo

The flavonol icarin present in Epimedium has been shown to improve circulation to the penis or clitoris by affecting nitric oxide pathways.[111] The plant is rich in constituents that are hormonally modulating, suggesting several mechanisms of action.

Traditionally, Epimedium has been found useful for fatigue, suggesting possible adaptogen activity. One writer describes this plant as dramatic in its ability to "boost essence" and stimulate kidney yang.[112,113,114]

Epimedium has also been used for menstrual irregularities and hypertension. Flavonoids lend anti-inflammatory, and antioxidant properties. As a neuroprotective agent, Epimedium helps improve memory and cognition and may alleviate symptoms of depression.[115,116] Constituents include flavonoids with icarin thought to be most active, sterols, sesquiterpenes, polysaccharides, and lignans.

Erythroxylum catuaba (Catuaba)

Another nervous system tonic with probable adaptogenic activity, Catuaba is perhaps the most famed of all Brazilian aphrodisiac herbs. The Indigenous people have many songs praising its virtues and it is said that if a man fathers a child before the age of 60, the child is his, but if he should father a child after turning 60, his progeny is considered the child of catuaba. (Taylor) Certainly with such a reputation as this, the plant cannot be ignored when treating men struggling with waning sexual function.

Other traditional uses include the treatment of nervous exhaustion, agitation, anxiety, poor memory and insomnia, all symptoms suggestive of possible adaptogenic activity.

Like potency wood, the plant has low toxicity. It also has antibacterial and antiviral activity.[108]

Turnera aphrodesiatica (Damiana)

A warming pelvic decongestant, damiana may be considered for urinary incontinence, amenorrhea, leucorrhea, dysmenorrhea, infertility, general nervousness, and fatigue. It is said to be stimulating, uplifting and invigorating.

Traditionally used in Mayan tradition as an aphrodisiac herb,[109] damiana is tonic to the reproductive hormonal system. Although the plant does contain some alkaloids that are similar to those found in Yohimbe, it does not appear to be as overly stimulating as Yohimbe, although some sources suggest long term use of damiana may not be wise due to stimulating qualities of the plant. Constituents include caffeine, arbutine, flavonoids, beta-sitosterol, tannin, and an essential oil.

Smilax officinalis (Sarsaparilla)

Rich in saponins and plant sterols, Smilax serves as a beneficial supportive herb in a formula for sexual dysfunction. Traditionally, the plant has been used for impotence, skin conditions, psoriasis, and rheumatism. Because the type of bacteria found in both syphilis and Lyme disease are spirochetes, the historical use of Smilax for the treatment of syphilis[110] suggests that Smilax should perhaps be considered as an adjunctive herb in the treatment of patients infected with the Borrelia spirochete (Lyme disease).

Smilax is an alterative and blood cleanser. It also has anti-inflammatory and hepato-protective activity. It is often included in women's formulas blended to support the luteal phase of the menstrual cycle, as it is thought to support progesterone metabolism.

Pedicularis spp.

Common to the Pacific Northwest, Pedicularis has been helpful in some cases of erectile dysfunction. It should be administered in milder cases before importing more exotic herbs from the Amazon. Flavonoids present in the plant give it anti-inflammatory and antioxidant activity and there is some suggestion that it may be useful as an anticancer agent. For more on this most excellent herb, see the chapter on musculo-skeletal herbs.

Eurycoma longifolia (Tongkal ali)

This Malasian herb has been shown to increase testosterone, sperm count, and libido. It is tonic to the reproductive tract and increases circulation and immune function. Although I have not used this particular herb, it is of note that it may be specifically helpful for decreasing premature ejaculations.

Tribulus terrestris (Puncture Vine)

Tribulus is another tonic herb that may help with erectile dysfunction. It is a common weed in parts of Asia and Europe. In addition to improving sexual function, Tribulus increases luteinizing hormone and testosterone, and improves fertility. It has antimicrobial and anti-tumor activity. As a cardiovascular medicine the plant may decrease high cholesterol levels and high blood pressure, as well as frequency of angina attacks in those patients already suffering from cardiac disease.

Constituents include steroidal saponins, with protodioscin considered to be the most active known constituent. It may also have some antioxidant properties.

Pausinystalia yohimbe (Yohimbe)

Although fairly well known for its ability to stimulate erectile function, this herb is often contraindicated in the very men who need it. Hypertension, increased heart rate, hot flashes, anxiety, and insomnia are all potential side effects, suggesting sympathetic nervous system stimulation with resultant cardiovascular stress. The herb is obviously contraindicated in hypertension or cardiovascular disease, or anyone with a tendency to anxiety. It is also contraindicated in diabetes, and liver and kidney disease. Foods rich in tyramine need to be avoided if taking this herb and the drug phenylpropylalanine, found in over the counter nasal decongestants, also needs to be avoided. Overdoses of yohimbe can be fatal.

Foods high in tyramine include, but are not limited to, many aged, fermented, processed, or pickled, meats and cheeses, chocolate, alcoholic beverages, soy sauce, miso, tempeh, broad leaf legumes such as fava beans, green beans, or snow peas. Many otherwise healthy foods such as avocades, raspberries, plums, coconut, figs and eggpant also contain significant amounts of tyramine. It may be best to choose another herb for sexual enhancement.

The alkaloid yohimbine is considered the active constituent.

When yohimbe is compared to the previously discussed herbs, many of which are nervines with adaptogenic activity, it is hard to even consider using this plant. However, it may be a valuable addition for stubborn cases when used in low doses to potentize a formula, and then only when it is not otherwise contraindicated. I have not found any need to use this herb in the men I have treated for erectile dysfunction.

Ginkgo biloba

As a general circulatory stimulant and flavonoid-rich anti-oxidant herb, gingko often appears in formulas for erectile dysfunction. For more about Ginkgo, see the chapter on cognitive dysfunction.

L-Arginine

Although I find that the herbs do an excellent job, the amino acid L-arginine is commonly used in treating erectile dysfunction. It appears to relax arterial tension via nitric oxide pathways, increasing blood flow to the arteries feeding sexual organs. It increases libido and has been used topically in creams to improve orgasm. As an arterial relaxant, arginine can also prove helpful in the treatment of hypertension and may help reduce elevated cholesterol levels.

Arginine is contraindicated in schizophrenia, infection with herpes virus, and diabetes.

A Few Final Words

Enhancing pelvic circulation by encouraging yoga postures, movement therapies, horesback riding, and/or kegel exercises are important to include as part of an overall protocol. Spinal fixations in the low back should also be addressed.

Chapter 17

Acute Urinary Tract Infections

ACUTE BLADDER INFECTIONS, known medically as urinary cystitis, do not usually require the use of anti-biotics. Mild symptoms often respond to increased fluids, extra Vitamin C, and unsweetened cranberry juice. More intense symptoms that do not respond to these simple measures nearly always do well with a homeopathic remedy, even when pain is intense or there is blood in the urine. The addition of herbs that are anti-microbial, demulcent, and disinfectant in the urinary tract help nourish and support the healing process.

Although any number of homeopathic remedies could be indicated, including the patient's constitutional remedy, there are a few remedies that usually serve to clear up an episode of acute cystitis.

Sarsaparilla is the most common homeopathic remedy for treating acute cystitis. Symptoms guiding us to choose this remedy include burning or cramping pain that is worse at the end of urination.

Staphysagria comes up when cystitis occurs after coition. Often there will be a tendency to bladder infections or urethritis after coition.

Although homeopathic Cantharis has acquired a reputation for treating cystitis, it does not seem to work as commonly as the other two remedies and I have only rarely found it useful. Better results are obtained with Sarsaparilla or Staphysagria.

If a patient comes to clinic with fever and chills and looking really weak and sick with a bladder infection then Pyrogen should be considered. I have only used this remedy a few times for cystitis over the years, but I have been glad to know of it when it was needed.

Like any acute, I go with a 30C every 2 - 4 hours or a 200C every 4 - 6 hours for the first 24 hours, with frequency of repetition dependent on severity of symptoms. Doses should be spaced further apart if symptoms begin to resolve. The important thing is to follow the symptoms.

Below is a group of herbs that can be formulated in tincture for cystitis.

Archtostaphylos uva ursi (Uva Ursi)
Chimaphila spp. (Pipsissewa, Prince's Pine)
Barosma betulina/Agathosma betulina (Buchu)
Agropyrum repens (Couch Grass)
Equisetum arvense (Horsetail)
Zea mays (Corn Silk)
Echinacea
Silica 6x

The formula works well when mixed with urinary disinfectants, Echinacea, and demulcents. It can be dosed at 60 drops every 2 hours for 2 days while awake then every 4 hours until symptoms are cleared. The formula should be continued 3 or 4 times per day for a few days after symptoms are gone.

A tea of some of the same herbs should also be given with at least 4 cups taken per day.

Uva ursi, a member of the Ericaceae family, is common the northwest forests and is often used in landscape design as a ground cover. Uva ursi is astringent, diuretic, disinfectant, and anti-microbial in the urinary tract. It can be irritating if used long term or in doses sufficient to clear a bladder infection on its own. I have never had any problem with using it over a few weeks or in frequent dosing for an acute infection, but that is probably because I never use it as a simple, but always in formula with other herbs, so that the dose of the one herb remains minimal.

Like uva ursi, Chimaphila, common name pipsissewa or prince's pine, is a member of the Ericaceae family. Chimaphila is diuretic, astringent, tonic and alterative. Unlike uva ursi, Chimaphila is gentle and appropriate for long term use.

Buchu is a member of the plant family Rutaceae. I do not always include it in my formulas for the simple reason that it must be imported from South Africa and our local herbs are quite efficacious. Buchu is anti-microbial, anti-inflammatory and diuretic.

The rhizome of couch grass is anti-microbial, demulcent, and diuretic. Both Chimaphila and couch grass have also been used for gout and rheumatic complaints.

The astringency of Equisetum arvense makes it especially useful when hematuria (blood in the urine) is present. It is also diuretic and cooling.

Zea mays is a soothing demulcent in the urinary tract.

The addition of Echinacea and homeopathic silica 6X to urinary tract tinctures has improved results significantly. Both act in different ways to support immune function.

Chapter 18
Hawthorne: Not Just a Cardiovascular Herb

THERE IS A SIGNIFICANT AMOUNT OF MODERN scientific research validating the efficacy of Crataegus spp. in the treatment of cardiovascular disease. A flavonoid-rich, nutritive tonic, hawthorne enhances cardiovascular health by decreasing inflammation, opening coronary vessels, lowering blood pressure, and generally strengthening the function and integrity of cardiovascular tissue. The anthocyanin-rich flavonoids present in berries and flowers provide anti-inflammatory and anti-oxidant activity and improve cross linkage in the connective tissue of blood vessels. By providing the nutritional foundation for a healthier heart and blood vessels, hawthorne enhances the actions of other therapies aimed at improving cardiovascular health.

The use of Crataegus should not be reserved solely for those patients with frank pathology. When taken periodically as a tea, tincture, or jam of the berries, hawthorne is an important food for keeping the cardiovascular system healthy.

The first time I had the privilege to meet this plant in nature, I was overwhelmed by the outpouring of unconditional love and bountiful generosity that opened and filled my unsuspecting heart. As I stepped between two branches dripping with an abundance of white spring blossoms, the tree poured a bounty of tender compassion into my heart, bringing tears to my eyes. I felt as if I was being cradled in the arms of my Divine Mother, protected and loved as I had never been loved before.

As a result of how touched I was by my initial encounter, I became entranced with the little tree and her gifts. Over the next several months, I began to cultivate a deeper relationship with the plant, going into nature as often as possible to be in her presence. I harvested blossoms in spring and berries in fall, from which I made teas, tinctures, and jam. In spring I made a flower essence from the blossoms, which I have since found invaluable in my practice. In addition, I spent every moment I could studying the old books and perusing the modern research. I added dried berries to the contents of the medicine bag I wore around my neck and carried a one-ounce bottle of tincture with me wherever I went, randomly taking drop doses and noting my response.

It was not long before I noticed a pattern emerge. Whether ingesting the tincture, tea, berries, solid extract, or flower essence, hawthorne, I discovered, gently helped keep my heart open when I would otherwise have closed down. If I was unconscious of an underlying grief or sadness, a few drops of the herb would cause the hidden emotion to gently bubble up for conscious processing, while a few drops taken in the midst of experiencing these same feelings would bring relief and lighten my heart.

I soon discovered, however, that this very wise plant did not intend for me to simply open my heart indiscriminately. Scattered among the fragrant white blossoms of spring, or the deep red berries of autumn, are sharp thorns that warn us to treat this generous member of the rose family with respect. In this way she teaches us that we must be willing to protect our compassionate open-heartedness and generosity, insisting on respect, even if it means speaking a bit sharply at times. If we humans could *re-member* respect for each other and all living things, the world would be a better place.

Perhaps the best time for using Crataegus as a nutritive tonic for the prevention of cardiovascular disease comes when life circumstances such as loss, grief, betrayal, trauma, or abuse, past or present, create the potential for us to close down emotionally. It may also be used to tonify the emotions for those patients who are either closed to their emotions or drowning in the enormity of grief. In these cases, hawthorne opens and cleanses the emotional heart, clearing acute or chronic emotional distress, as surely as she opens the coronary arteries in cases of acute angina.

One young woman whose heart was full of rage and jealousy at another family member was given homeopathic Lachesis and a preparation of hawthorne to be taken 1/4 teaspoon four times per day. The frequency of four times per day was recommended to awaken the 4th chakra energy. On the follow-up visit her rage at her sister was thankfully gone, most likely from the effects of the Lachesis, but throughout the visit she kept repeating, "Oh, I just love that hawthorne!"

"What is it that you love so much about the hawthorne?" I queried her.

"Oh!" she replied enthusiastically. "It just opens my heart and I feel such warmth inside. You know people are really not so bad."

Another woman who had silently suffered from a lifelong suicidal depression found resolution of symptoms after taking homeopathic Aurum. At her third follow-up, I began to think about how reluctant and closed she was in sharing her emotions, and although her depression was gone, she was still overly serious and solemn in her demeanor. I decided to try adding some hawthorne to her herbal antidepressant formula.

Refilling her tincture of borage, black cohosh, and hypericum, I added just enough hawthorne to give her the equivalent of one drop per dose of tincture four times per day.

On follow-up a few weeks later, not only was she no longer depressed, she was exuberant. I was astonished at the excitement and joy that emanated from her.

"Dr. Frances," she kept repeating throughout the visit. "Don't take that new herb from me! Please promise you won't take that new herb from me!"

The depression never returned. Even many years later, when significant stressors entered her life, there was not the slightest sign of the depression she had once endured for so long.

On one occasion, while listening to a holistic veterinarian give a talk at an herb conference, tears of grief welled up as I thought of my little Peruvian mare, Rosa, who had endured so much suffering as a result of developing a severe neurological disease. I had treated Rosa with intensive prescribing of herbs and homeopathy, and although she had recovered, the stress and grief I felt at seeing her so ill for the better part of a year, had been pushed aside so I could take charge and deal with her illness. The veterinarian's lecture brought out a much-needed emotional discharge, but as I was scheduled to lecture in the same room immediately after her, I felt some necessity to pull myself together. Following the lecture, I retired to the restroom to wash my face in cold water. I added a few deep breaths and felt fine. On returning to the room to prepare for my lecture, however, I made the mistake of asking the folks who were just filing in,

"Did any of you hear that last lecture with the veterinarian?"

Well that was it. The faucet opened full force and now the tears were absolutely unstoppable.

As luck would have it, I had ordered several bottles of hawthorne tincture to pass around for people to experience during the lecture, so I grabbed a bottle from the box in front of me and took a dropperful, then another and another. With each dose I could feel a huge layer of grief and sadness lift from my chest but it took nearly half the bottle before I was coherent. A bit of laughter bubbled up through my tears at the absurdity of my position. Without apologizing for my grief, I shared a bit of my mare's story.

"Oh well," I said with a shrug of surrender to the process. "I guess I'll just lecture through the tears!"

I was only a few moments into the lecture when the hawthorne I had been guzzling had finally lifted enough of the grief that the tears could stop flowing. As the lecture progressed, the 75 people who filled the room radiated a softer more receptive energy than I have ever experienced in my many years of teaching. As we passed herbs around for tasting, participants were more open in sharing their experiences, perhaps feeling that their vulnerabilities were less likely to be judged in a class where the instructor was comfortable with the flow of emotion.

Hawthorne can also be helpful for patients who are closed to loving themselves or parts of their human nature. One patient who would not open to his fiery side, despite dream images that encouraged him to so, remained a stubborn doormat, allowing others to push him around rather than take his power and stand up for himself. After a serious bout of pneumonia, he turned up at my clinic with a thoracic fixation that would not yield, or if it did, would seize up again within the week. I had prescribed a good formula of the anti-spasmodic and anti-inflammatory herbs that worked so reliably most of the time, dosing them generously and often, but to no avail. As I came to know a bit more about him, I began to suspect that the bout of pneumonia and persistent thoracic fixation were related to his inability to open to the beauty of his sacred warrior side. I prescribed a tincture of hawthorne to be taken four times per day with the hope that he might be able to open his heart to his more fiery side and integrate his power. On the next visit, the patient appeared more relaxed. The vertebra was easily released, remaining mobile after the visit for the first time. In the months that followed, he was able to realize the value of claiming his fire and standing up for himself and those that he loved.

In the old literature, there are a few references to the use of hawthorne in emotional states. Benedict Lust says that hawthorne is useful for "nervous conditions, particularly insomnia" and the Eclectic physician Ellingwood tells us "It dispels gloomy forbodings...(and) causes a general sense of well being."

It was not long before I began to realize that the emotions for which hawthorne was proving so beneficial, were the same emotional states that are related to the lungs. I began to wonder if the herb would be as helpful for lung conditions when the same symptoms of tightness and constriction or heaviness in the chest that called for its use in cardiac conditions manifested as part of a bronchial or lung condition.

The Universe, in its great generosity, soon gifted me with a bout of acute bronchitis accompanied by chest tightness and constriction. I made up a respiratory formula of soothing, demulcent, and expectorant herbs and started myself on homeopathic Kali carbonicum 200C. All of this was moving the healing process along quite nicely, but when the constriction worsened, suggesting that a repeat of the remedy was in order, I reached for the hawthorne instead, placing four drops of the tincture straight onto my tongue. To my astonishment the response was immediate. My chest opened up, the tightness and constriction disappeared instantly, my breathing eased, and I began to perspire over both my chest and back.

Shortly after this experience I began dispensing hawthorne tincture as a simple for asthma, instructing patients to take a full dropperful every minute or so as needed for dyspnea (difficulty breathing) or whenever they felt the need to reach for their inhaler. Assuring them that the herb has been used for centuries as a food and is completely nontoxic, I directed them to repeat the dose as often as needed, even every _ to 1 minute if necessary. If after five doses they were still symptomatic, I told them they then had my permission to use their inhaler. This protocol is always prescribed in conjunction with my usual regimen of constitutional homeopathy and other herbal formulas to support the lungs, immune system, and adrenal cortex. In addition, dairy products and other possible allergens are removed from the diet.

To my astonishment, patients were returning for their three week follow up appointments completely off their inhalers. Although I had always suggested other bronchodilating herbs, including Ephedra sinensis, for acute use in asthma, I had never seen such remarkable results so quickly.

The large majority of asthma cases are of atopic origin in which a hypersensitivity response to an external stimulus creates an inflammatory reaction in the bronchial tree resulting in coughing, wheezing, dyspnea, and a prolonged expiratory phase of respiration. Pathophysiology includes the release of multiple primary and secondary mediators of inflammation, including mast cells, basophils, lymphocytes, macrophages and eosinophils. Histamine release from mast cells and basophils may be one of the most important mediators in the onset of acute symptoms, resulting in acute bronchospasm, increased vascular permeability and increased bronchial secretions. Platelet activating factor (PAF), also released from mast cells, and IgE sensitized basophils further contribute to increased vascular permeability in the bronchial tree. Cellular release of prostaglandins (PGD2) and leukotrienes (LT, C4, D4, E4) contribute to bronchoconstriction and further increase in vascular permeability. Free radicals create epithelial tissue damage, adding to the overall picture of wheezing, dyspnea, and bronchospasm.

Crataegus is high in a number of flavonoids, including anthocyanins, proanthocyanadins, quercitin, quercitin-3-galactoside, vitexin, and vitexin-4-rhamnoside.[117] Many of these compounds have been shown to stabilize collagen matrix, thereby strengthening blood vessel walls, leading to a decrease in capillary fragility and vascular permeability. Several of these flavonoids also act to inhibit the release of secondary mediators of inflammation from leukocytes, such as leukotrienes and prostaglandins.

Most of my patients have reported immediate relief after the first dose or two of the medicine, rarely needing to go beyond three doses. This suggests that while all the biochemistry is validating and of definite interest in the treatment of allergic asthma, an energetic, "Heart Chakra" response is also at play in the dramatic improvement of acute symptomotology.

In the years that followed it was only the occasional asthma patient that did not respond to the use of hawthorne for their asthma. Two highly cerebral men, one with

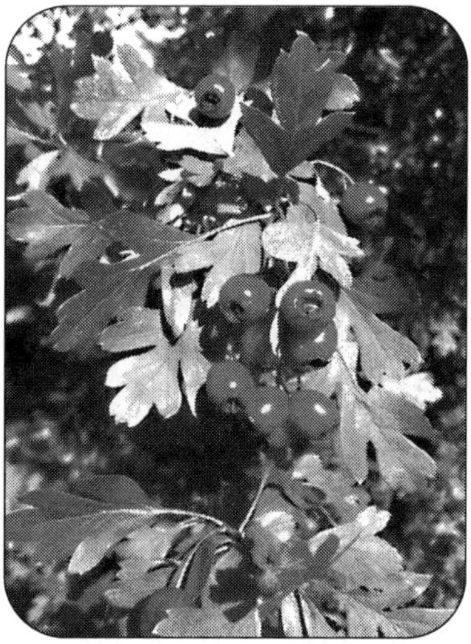

Hawthorne
Photo courtesy of Orna Izakson N.D.

asthma and another with chronic obstructive pulmonary disease, which also usually responds very nicely to the use of Crataegus, did better with osha (Ligusticum porteri). To my surprise, both of these very proper business men took great delight in carrying a piece of osha root in their shirt pockets and bringing it out in the office amongst their colleagues whenever shortness of breath called for its use. I instructed them to chew on the end of the root then inhale deeply to take the essential oils into their lungs. This invariably brought relief to these two "heady" fellows who needed a root to ground them, rather than the flower or berry of the hawthorne.

As osha is in danger of being overharvested, I prefer to reserve its use for those who need just that herb. Hawthorne, however, is easily grown and effortlessly supplies us with generous amounts of both berries and flowers.

It is important to remember that patients taking steroid-containing inhalers regularly should always wean use of their inhalers gradually to avoid a rebound effect.

Although I have been using hawthorne for asthma for a good 20 years in clinical practice, it is only recently that I have been able to discover any reference in the scientific literature to the use of hawthorne for respiratory conditions. A study published in 2012, a good twenty years from the date I began using it for asthma, reveals that hawthorne may be useful in the treatment of allergic airway disease.[118]

Hawthorne can also be used as a simple for the treatment of acute angina, a more time-honored use. A dropperful of tincture is taken as needed for chest pain with permission to resort to sublingual nitroglycerine (the drug commonly prescribed to dilate coronary blood vessels) if symptom relief is not obtained within 3 - 5 doses. Patients are often very glad to find a substitute for the nitroglycerine as the drug dilates vessels in the head as well as the heart, often leaving patients with a headache. If chest pain does not respond to either hawthorne or nitroglycerine, medical care should be sought immediately to assure that the patient is not experiencing a heart attack.

Hawthorne will increase blood flow to the brain if indicated, but unlike the nitroglycerine used for angina, it will not do so to the point of causing headache. One patient who was experiencing a sudden onset of confusion and amnesia was given a solid extract of hawthorne to eat by the teaspoon on the way to the emergency room. By the time she and her daughter arrived at the hospital, she was already feeling better, and later reported that her symptoms diminished dose by dose from the first each teaspoon of hawthorne she ingested. She was given the diagnosis of transient ischemic attack, commonly called "mini-stroke" at the hospital.

A native Irish herbalist recently informed me that in Ireland, where hawthorne is still considered sacred, it is said that bad luck will come to any who cuts down a hawthorne tree. For that reason many fields where other trees have been cleared to allow planting will have the occasional tree standing alone in the middle of the field. That tree is inevitably a hawthorne. Hawthorne is central to Celtic spiritual practices and there are also stories that the crown of thorns worn by Jesus during his crucifixion was hawthorne.

Functional Heart Palpitations:

Linden, Leonurus, and Passiflora

In these high stress times, herbal nervines play a vital role in restoring and maintaining health. These three nervines affect the heart center in different but complimentary ways, and all are useful in the treatment of functional heart palpitations. For more on Leonurus, Passiflora, and Tilia, see the chapter on nervines.

Linden Flower (Tilia spp.) Tiliaceae

For those gloomy moments that life occasionally, or not so occasionally, sends our way, Tilia brings its dancing spirit to lighten our hearts and chase away the blues. Its adaptogenic and blood purifying qualities combine to help us cope with the stressors that led us to fall into the blues in the first place. Because I have consistently seen such remarkable results with Leonurus, I have never used Tilia for functional heart palpitations, but the old books suggest it may be of service in these patients. Combining Tilia's uplifting, adaptogenic, nervine, blood cleansing, antispasmodic, and antihypertensive properties with its affinity for the cardiovascular system certainly makes it a good candidate for the job.

Dosage for a tincture of Tilia is 60 drops 3 times per day or 40 drops 4 times per day.

Motherwort (Leonurus cardiaca) Lamiaceae

In her role as a nervine, motherwort calms the cardiac plexus as well as the central nervous system. As such, she is the plant of choice for men or women struggling with functional heart palpitations. Although these symptoms, which include irregular, thumping heart beats or racing high heart rates, can often be frightening, they are usually not life threatening. Arising in the absence of organic cardiac disease, functional heart palpitations are usually associated with stress. In fact, the anxiety that is so frequently blamed for the occurrence of palpitations is often due to physiologic stress, such as toxicity, poor digestion, or the hormonal stress of menopause. In her great wisdom, Leonurus addresses all of these factors. Calming nervine properties combine with bitter constituents that stimulate stagnant liver and digestive function, while other properties of the plant blend to tone the reproductive system, improving circulation to the pelvis and easing hormonal tension. Flavonoids present in the plant join to decrease inflammation and toxicity.

Functional heart palpitations often respond well to a tincture that includes equal parts of Leonurus and Crataegus, dosed 30 to 60 drops three times per day.

Passionflower (Passiflora incarnate) Passifloraceae

Although I find Leonurus to be our most reliable medicine for the treatment of functional heart palpitations, Passiflora is also indicated for palpitations, especially when symptoms are due to lack of sleep or general anxiety and tension, particularly when stresses result in emotional heartache. It is a specific sedative nervine for the heartfelt or emotional constitution.

Both passionflower and motherwort are discussed in more detail in the chapter on nervines.

Chapter 19
Hypertension

HYPERTENSION IS CONSIDERED A SIGNIFICANT RISK FACTOR in the development of cardiovascular disease and can also be a direct cause of renal failure. Causes of hypertension are often multifaceted, but the buildup of atherosclerotic plaque with the resultant reduced flexibility of vessel walls and increase in inflammation are still considered important etiologic mechanisms for high blood pressure. Stress and chronic nervous tension also contribute to increased blood pressure. Renal disease must be ruled out as an underlying cause, especially if blood pressure is unresponsive to therapy and/or dangerously elevated. Renal disease can also occur due to longstanding hypertension.

Hypertension is usually asymptomatic, although the rare person will complain of symptoms when their blood pressure spikes to elevated levels. Such symptoms may include headaches, a pulsing sensation in the body synchronous with heart beat, or a flushed face.

The top number in blood pressure readings, called the systolic blood pressure, is a measurement of the arterial pressure when the ventricles of the heart are actively contracting to push blood from the heart into the vessels. This first number is generally more influenced by stress than the lower number, which is known as the diastolic blood pressure. Diastolic readings are a measurement of arterial pressure when the heart is at rest. Although both readings are important, elevations in diastolic blood pressure are generally considered more critical. Not realizing the importance of diastolic blood pressure, patients often report only the top, systolic blood pressure reading.

It is wise to remember that one blood pressure reading does not make a diagnosis. As readings are often higher when taken during an office visit, it is best to have patients bring in several readings from home and look at the general trend. This practice also prevents the practitioner from treating "white coat hypertension", a phenomenon where blood pressure is elevated only in the physician's office. In addition, a blood pressure diary makes evaluation of treatment more precise, as follow-up readings are gauged against a more accurate baseline.

Although there has been some discussion about changing the criteria for the diagnosis of hypertension, the classification I use for evaluating blood pressure is as follows:

Borderline Hypertension: 120 - 140 / 85 - 90
Mild Hypertension: 140 - 160 / 90 - 100
Moderate Hypertension: 160 - 180 / 100 - 115
Severe Hypertension: 180+ / 115+

Because naturopathic medicine offers safe, non-toxic modalities for the treatment of hypertension, I usually initiate treatment whenever blood pressure is persistently over 140/85 with the hope of arresting further progression. Hopefully the last chapter will have informed the reader that the first herb to use for initiating treatment is Crataegus (hawthorne). The nutritive and cardiovascular protective actions of hawthorne make it important in creating a foundation that increases efficacy of any other therapies. Although Crataegus may help as a single medicinal agent in the treatment of early-onset mild hypertension, more often it does its best work by acting synergistically with other herbs.

This synergistic effect has also been observed when patients are concurrently taking pharmaceutical medications, particularly beta blockers. In these cases, the addition of Crataegus may allow for reduced dosing of pharmaceuticals, or discontinuance althogether.

Close attention to nutrition, encouraging a wide variety of fresh fruits and vegetables with an emphasis on plenty of garlic, celery, dark green leafy vegetables and fresh fruits is vital.

If a simple of hawthorne and dietary measures are not adequate in bringing down blood pressure, Tilia (linden flower) should be the next herb to consider.

Although severe hypertension or very stubborn cases may require stronger medicines, Tilia is often highly effective when readings are only moderately elevated. Its anti-spasmodic, anti-atherosclerotic, vaso-dilating, diaphoretic, and diuretic properties all combine to contribute to its effectiveness as an anti-hypertensive.

As a calming, uplifting nervine, Tilia may act as a helpful adjunct in healing the nervous system in patients who struggle with anxiety and depression. It also possesses some activity as an adrenal adaptogen, mitigating the effects of chronic stress, emotionally as well as physically. It is efficacious as an anti-viral herb where it has been used in the treatment and prevention of colds. A hot tea would undoubtedly amplify the diaphoretic effects, further enhancing the plant's antiviral properties. Indigestion due to a nervous stomach, nervous vomiting, and migraines may all be helped by the addition of Tilia. It is also a blood purifier.

For diaphoretic effects or as an antiviral, a hot infusion of leaf and flower, 1 - 2 teaspoons per cup, may be preferred. The tincture (1:5 dry) can be given at 15 - 40 drops 2 - 4 times per day. It may also be used in a bath to soothe an overwrought nervous system. Here the neutral bath would be preferable. (See chapter on nervines for more information on the neutral bath).

Constituents include a volatile oil, tannins, mucilage, and glycosides.

Tilia is also useful for treating arrhythmias related to stress. In these cases it is important to remove simple sugars from the diet before initiating herbal therapies for the treatment of cardiac arrhythmia.

One patient who suffered from frequent PVCs after a heart attack, (PVCs are premature ventricular contractions, a type of cardiac arrythmia that can be serious for patients who have had a heart attack), experienced complete resolution of his arrhythmia after taking the enormous amount of sugar he was in the habit of ingesting out of his diet. Although hawthorne was given to feed and nourish the heart, he did not require intensive herbal treatment for his cardiac symptoms.

Other plants that can prove supportive in formulas for hypertension include, Achillea millefolium, (yarrow flowers) which acts as a peripheral vasodilator and anti-inflammatory, and Actea/Cimicifuga racemosa (black cohosh) which is anti-spasmodic to vessel walls, anti-inflammatory, and also acts as an anti-depressant nervine.

Despite its relatively high sodium content, Apium graveolens (celery), will often prove helpful in lowering blood pressure. It is rich in magnesium, potassium and calcium, all of which are supportive of healthy cardiovascular function. Ingestion of four stalks of celery a day adds a diuretic action. This plant is contraindicated in patients with kidney disease. The leaf of the common dandelion, Taraxacum officinalis, is another excellent diuretic for use in hypertension. Other diuretic herbs that may be of help include Galium aparine, Juniperus berries, Equisetum arvense, Uva ursi, and the leaves of Urtica dioica. Tilia and Crataegus are also diuretic

The beautiful, lusciously red hibiscus flowers, Hibiscus spp., are full of flavonoids known as anthocyanins and make a colorful, tasty tea. Hibiscus will lower systolic blood pressure, but may not prove as helpful in bringing down diastolic readings. The plant is calming to the nervous system, anti-spasmodic and diruetic.

Scutellaria lateriflora (skullcap) and Viburnum opulus (cramp bark) are both hypotensive via anti-spasmodic mechanisms. Viburnum also has anti-inflammatory activity while both plants act as nervines to soothe and nourish the nervous system.

Melissa officinalis (lemon balm) is vasodilating, anti-oxidant and mildly anti-spasmodic in its hypotensive actions. Melissa is also a calming nervine with some uplifting properties as well.

Passiflora incarnata (Passiflora) and Valeriana spp. (Valerian) are both sedative nervines that possess anti-spasmodic and hypotensive activity. Passiflora is anti-inflammatory.

Viscum album, the European mistletoe, contains bitters, mucilage, tannins, a fixed oil and a resin known as viscin. Low doses are mildly hypotensive over the long term while higher doses raise blood pressure. (Felter) The herb acts to reduce hypertension by several mechanisms, including vasodilation of peripheral vessels, and nervine and para-sympathomimetic acivity. Viscum is specifically indicated for the patient with a flushed face, tendency to congestive headaches, irritability and dizziness.

Viscum also strengthens cardiac contractility, resulting in more efficient cardiac muscle contraction with improved cardiac output. It is soothing to oversensitive cardiac nerves, producing a decrease in arrhythmias. It is also indicated for valvular insufficiency, cardiac hypertrophy, and a weak irregular pulse.

Viscum is tonic to both gastro-intestinal and genitor-urinary tracts. This effect may be at least partially due to stimulation of parasympathetic activity resulting in a shunting of blood and nutrients to these vital organ systems. It has been used for the treatment of rheumatic conditions and neuralgia. The plant acts as a muscular relaxant and anti-convulsant in small doses, although large doses have the opposite effect causing increased muscle spasm and convulsions.

Although very safe for long-term use in proper doses, Viscum is a potentially toxic plant and generally only available to licensed health care practitioners. Symptoms of toxicity include nausea and vomiting, bloody diarrhea, contracted pupils, tetanus, convulsions, hallucinations, coma, and ultimately death via cardiovascular collapse. A 1:5 tincture may generally be dosed at 1 - 15 drops one to four times daily. (Tilgner)

The root of Veratrum viride, green hellebore, also a low-dose botanical generally only available to licensed healthcare practitioners, is much more rapid acting than Viscum in bringing down blood pressure. Although it can be a useful adjunct in antihypertensive herbal formulas dosed four times per day, small frequent dosing of this plant may be more efficacious, as its action is rapid and short lived and it is rapidly excreted from the body. When frequent repetition is practical or necessary, the full 24-hour dose of tincture can be mixed in a quart of drinking water and sipped throughout the day. Such dosing should only be done under the supervision of a qualified health care provider who can monitor for potential toxicity and hypotension.

Veratrum is specific for the patient who presents with a flushed face, full bounding pulse with a hard ropy quality, and a sensation of pulsation in the ears. The herb slows heart and respiratory rates and is anti-inflammatory. Constituents include several alkaloids and a resin. Like most potentially toxic plants, the first indications of overdose with Veratrum are nausea and vomiting, nature's way of protecting us from further danger. More progressive symptoms include diarrhea, gastric and pharyngeal burning, sneezing, lachrymation and salivation, a weak racing pulse, dizziness, fainting, hypotension, shock, cold clammy diaphoresis, decreased body temperature, dilated pupils, and finally respiratory arrest.

With medical supervision, the plant can be dosed as high as 1 - 10 drops every 2 - 4 hours for the treatment of acute hypertensive crises, decreasing doses if signs of toxicity appear. Smaller doses can be added to formulas as a synergist to potentize the formula.

Garlic is well known for its ability to reduce blood pressure. It is also diuretic, hepatoprotective, and anti-coagulant. Garlic is an excellent anti-parasitic and anti-microbial agent. Where it was once used to ward off bad spirits, garlic now finds fame for warding off colds, flu, and other infections … different ways of saying the same thing. Garlic is most effective when used fresh and raw.

Garlic Vinegar Recipe

1) Place raw crushed garlic in a glass jar.
2) Cover with enough good quality, apple cider vinegar to completely cover the garlic then heat to a boil. This step is necessary to kill the culture when raw vinegar is used.
3) Pour apple cider vinegar over the garlic until all garlic is covered.
4) Let the mixture sit in a cool dark place for 2 to 6 weeks, shaking or stirring daily.
5) After 2 to 6 weeks, garlic can be strained off and the vinegar may be used on salads or taken in juice or water. The garlic that has been strained off can be used in cooking or added raw to salads.

One quarter to one half teaspoon of the vinegar can be taken daily for cardiovascular effects or to prevent colds and flu. Doses may be increased to 4 times per day at the first sign of a respiratory infection.

Salvia miltiorrhiza (Chinese sage root) is a Chinese herb that is highly efficacious at normalizing glomerular function when kidneys are stressed. It has proven very effective in clinic for increasing abnormally low glomerular filtration rates (GFR). The herb is protective to the liver and kidneys,[119] tonic to cardiac tissue, and hypotensive.

Vinca minor (lesser periwinkle) may also be included in formulas for hypertension. It should not be confused with Vinca major which does not share the same cardiovascular effects. For more on Vinca minor see the next chapter on cognitive decline.

Rauwolfia serpentina, native to India, is one of our most effective agents in reducing blood pressure, particularly when milder herbs are not delivering the desired results. This plant is best reserved for cases with significantly elevated blood pressure or when other therapies prove inadequate. In the latter case, best results will be achieved when Rauwolfia is added to other therapies outlined above.

Rauwolfia works via neurotransmitter and catecholamine inhibition resulting in lowered blood pressure and decreased anxiety. Although here in the west Rauwolfia is used exclusively for the treatment of hypertension, it has historical use in India as a relaxing and sedative herb for tension, anxiety, and insomnia and as an antipsychotic[120]. Rauwolfia also has anti-arrhythmic activity, reduces the heart rate, and stimulates intestinal peristalsis.

Although the plant has over 50 known alkaloids, it acquired a bad reputation when medical practitioners in the early 20th century began to use the isolated alkaloid reserpine to treat high blood pressure. Side effects of severe depression were seen due to reserpine's tendency to deplete neurotransmitters that affect serotonin and dopamine. The drug (known as Serpasil) fell out of favor, as did the plant from which it was extracted. Nature's medicines, when respected and used appropriately, are generally far superior to isolated plant compounds. Other alkaloids in Rauwolfia have uplifting and euphoric qualities that balance the depressive nature of the reserpine, once again illustrating the wise blending and balancing of whole plant medicine versus standardized extracts.

Kenneth Proefrock N.D. (Arizona) and Yvon Rochon (owner of Herbal Vitality in Sedona, Arizona) have also worked with Rauwolfia vomitoria, which according to their research, has less of the reserpine and more of the calming and sedating alkaloids. Dr. Proefrock uses equal parts of R. serpentina and R. vomitoria in his treatment of hypertensive patients.[121]

I reserve the use of Rauwolfia for patients with moderate to severe hypertension or for those patients who are not responding optimally to other aforementioned therapies.

Cimicifuga/Actea racemosa, decreases blood pressure via antispasmodic and anti-inflammatory actions within blood vessel walls. This plant combines well with Rauwolfia, as it acts through a separate mechanism and adds additional antidepressant activity. In clinical practice, depression is rarely a concern, although it is wise to be cautious and monitor all patients newly starting on Rauwolfia.

Finally, stubborn cases will be helped by the addition of homeopathic Belladonna in low potency, such 3X, 3C, 6X, or 6C. Pellets can be added right into the herbal tincture, which should then be dosed 3 - 4 times per day.

As patients improve and BP readings stabilize, the homeopathic belladonna is discontinued first then Rauwolfia is tapered and discontinued as tolerated. I have generally found that I am not able to decrease the Rauwolfia for at least a couple years in most cases, so be patient. The hawthorne should be continued on and off for life as a nourishing preventative tonic.

Case

A 59 year old woman reported to clinic with a chief complaint of severe depression that had been going on for 5 - 7 years and was gradually getting worse. The depression had been creeping in for some time and she was unable to tie it to any specific stressor. She was in business for herself, running a very successful retail store for several years, which she had previously enjoyed. Although she admitted to thoughts of suicide, she was not actively suicidal. She also reported some mild asthmatic symptoms and a tendency to constipation.

On physical exam her blood pressure was elevated at 194/102.

"Yes I know it's really high," she said when we inquired about prior readings. "I am just too tired and depressed to do anything about it. It's terrible but I just don't have the energy to take care of myself like I should. It's not a bit like me. I am usually a real go-getter."

Her depression had prevented her from taking action with her blood pressure or changing her diet which was high in carbohydrates, sweets, and fried foods.

She was given homeopathic Aurum in an LM - 1 potency to be taken twice per day to address her depression and an herbal formula for hypertension that focused on herbs such as Cimicifuga/Actea and Tilia, to relieve depression. Achillea and Taraxacum were also included in the formula for liver support as hepatic congestion can often cause or aggravate depression. Crataegus was given in solid extract at doses of 1/2 teaspoon twice daily, also in part to address the depression. Although normally Rauwolfia would be included in a blood pressure formula for moderate to severely elevated blood pressure it was omitted from this patient's formula due to the severity of her depression.

While being sensitive to her inability to motivate herself due to the depression, dietary recommendations were shared, emphasizing fresh fruits and vegetables, high quality proteins and avoidance of fried and carbohydrate rich foods. It was also recommended that she consider discontinuing milk products and possibly gluten, given her tendency to asthmatic wheezing.

On follow-up 3 weeks later, the patient reported that the depression was gone.

"I can't believe it!" she exclaimed. "Can that homeopathic medicine really do that!? Even the asthma and constipation have disappeared!"

With the depression gone, her energy and motivation to care for herself had returned so she was able to improve her diet, although she was still eating gluten and wheat.

Her blood pressure diary revealed no change, with readings running from 180 - 210/92 - 104, but because the patient was now more motivated to address her hypertension, a product called Vasotensin, containing a peptide from the fish, bonito, was also dispensed with instructions to take 2 tabs twice per day. This product, available to physicians from Metagenics, has been shown to lower blood pressure, ostensibly via ACE inhibition.[122] A fish oil supplement was also recommended, but I continued to hold off with the Rauwolfia due to concerns about her depression.

Looking back I should have added Belladonna 6C into her herbal tincture since her blood pressure was so elevated and I was still reluctant to add in the Rauwolfia, but for some reason I did not think of it. Had I remembered, her blood pressure may have decreased without Rauwolfia.

Two weeks later, there was still no change in her blood pressure readings, so after discussing the options with her, we decided to add the Rauwolfia in and increase her Aurum to an LM - 2.

"If your depression threatens to return," I counseled her. "Call me and we will stop the Rauwolfia, but I honestly think you will be OK. There are more euphoria producing alkaloids in the whole plant than depressive ones."

On the next visit, again three weeks later, her blood pressure readings were much better, averaging 160 - 170/82 - 94. Her depression did not return despite the addition of Rauwolfia. Her blood pressure continued to normalize and within a few weeks she reported readings of 118 - 130/74 - 82.

Impressed with the results of her treatment, she finally decided to stop the gluten as we had recommended, "just to see." A couple months later, she brought her grandson in for an appointment and reported on her progress.

"I stopped gluten and was able to discontinue everything without any increase in blood pressure!"

"Great!" I responded. "Wheat and gluten seem to be coming up as culprits for some folks with hypertension. I am glad you were able to stop it."

"So am I!" she agreed joyfully.

Most of us feel that the problems people are having with wheat and gluten stem more from genetic mutations of the grains than from personal susceptibility. In years past, I almost never removed gluten or wheat from the diets of my patients, but now most of my patients are finding that they do better off gluten. The farther we move from nature the more we create problems, problems sadly evident in the genetic modification of our foods, which is wrecking havoc in people's health.

Chapter 20

Early Cognitive Dysfunction & Other Conditions Associated with Aging

MUCH OF THE SYMPTOMOTOLOGY commonly associated with the aging process is not necessarily a normal effect of aging. Symptoms such as cognitive decline, cataracts, osteoporosis, and others, while certainly widespread, are not inevitably intrinsic to the process of living longer. There is an odd tendency among medical professionals and the general populace to adopt an attitude of resignation to what is common, accepting it as normal and inevitable. This is an important point, because our perception of a problem directly affects how we relate to that problem. If we believe that any given health issue is just a normal part of being alive, we often surrender to a situation that can actually be changed.

I see many illustrations of this in daily practice, especially in association with symptoms that arise in aging, menopause, and in younger women in relation to their menstrual cycles. A common example is the assumed normalcy of premenstrual breast tenderness, a frequently occuring condition of lymphatic congestion in breast tissue which often responds well to a few simple dietary changes and herbal treatment, specifically with Ceanothus spp. tincture, taken 15 drops 3 times a day throughout the month. I am continually confronted with women who are surprised to discover that their premenstrual breast tenderness is not normal and that, in fact, some women don't experience it at all.

Decline in mental function at any age can be caused or exacerbated by poor diet, heavy metal toxicity, liver congestion, adrenal exhaustion, poor sleep habits, lack of exercise, thyroid dysfunction, blood sugar imbalances, and cardiovascular disease. Immune dysfunction, as is seen with allergies, auto immune disease, and chronic fatigue syndrome, can also contribute to decreased cognitive function. Depression, anxiety, grief, or other significant life stressors can also adversely affect cognition.

Isolation also affects cognitive ability. It has been well established that people who have a supportive network of friends, family, or animals in their lives have been shown to heal faster and remain healthier than people who live more isolated lives. Although we can't measure it in a test tube or inject it into laboratory rats for experimental purposes, love is a great healer.

Many of the toxins in our modern world are known to be damaging to the nervous system. Given this fact, how much of the cognitive difficulty we experience is really a normal part of aging? How much of the nervous system symptomatology we experience and witness in our patients is more accurately a symptom of a world no longer in touch with the beauty and sacredness of all life?

People who suffer from severe environmental sensitivity often report symptoms of nervous system dysfunction when exposed to chemical triggers. In these cases mental symptoms of agitation, depression, cloudy thinking, difficulty in focusing, and easy distractibility are due to congested detoxification pathways.

Cognitive changes are common in menopausal women but are not necessarily all normal. Although some shift to the more diffuse right brain, intuitive thinking is normal during menopause, liver congestion, adrenal exhaustion and heavy metal toxicity may have more to do with cognitive symptoms in menopause than menopause itself.

As with any chronic condition, treatment should be of a constitutional nature, individualized to each person's issues and healthcare needs. Assessment of liver, endocrine, cardiovascular, and immune function are fundamental. Treatment of cognitive declince specifically aimed at nourishing and healing the central nervous system will not be as effective without addressing other underlying health issues.

Treatment of Cognitive Dysfunction

A good B complex with minerals and antioxidants provides a basic nutritional foundation for optimal health at multiple levels. Most patients with cognitive dysfunction will also be helped by the addition of vitamin B12 as methylcobalamin 3000 - 6000 micrograms a day by mouth. For severe cases or for those patients who are not absorbing vitamin B12, which is often the case with older patients, or patients who are hypochlorhydric, 1000 micrograms may be given as an intramuscular injection 1 - 3 times a week, tapering down to once every week or two as symptoms improve. It may be wise to evaluate B12 status and establish a baseline prior to instituting therapy. A complete blood count (CBC) may show a high or high normal MCV on differential if a B12 deficiency exists. Serum B12 levels may be run but are rarely conclusive. A more recent test, methyl malonic acid is somewhat more expensive but may be more definitive in evaluating B12 status.

Although essential fatty acids (EFAs) are a vital part of any treatment program involving cognitive decline, excessive dosing of oils may increase risk for hemorrhagic incidents. The American public is woefully deficient in EFAs overall, which may be a contributing factor in the etiology of cognitive decline at any age. Flax oil at 1 tablespoon per day, and/or 1-2 teaspoons of cod liver or other fish oil may be considered. Other fish oil or supplements may provide higher doses of DHA than cod liver oil. DHA has specifically been shown to be beneficial in brain functioning.[123,124]

Medium chain triglycerides (MCTs) present in coconut oil have been shown to be instrumental in improving cognitive function.[125] Virgin and preferably organic coconut oil should be used with doses starting at 1 teaspoon with each meal, slowly working up to as much as 4 - 6 tablespoons per day.[126] Not everyone will require high dosing and care should be taken as intestinal cramping and diarrhea may occur if doses are increased too quickly. The oil should be incorporated into the diet as much as possible.

A tablespoon of organic, non GMO, lecithin, taken 1 - 3 times a day, supplies phosphotidylcholine which in turn provides the precursor, choline for the production of the neurotransmitter acetylcholine. In Alzheimer patients, the enzyme acetylcholine transferase, necessary for choline to bond to the acetyl molecule and create acetylcholine, has been shown to be deficient, thus creating an insufficient pool of the neurotransmitter acetylcholine.[127] Theoretically at least, supplementation of choline in the form of lecithin may be helpful by saturating what enzyme is present with plenty of raw material (choline) to form acetylcholine. Further studies are needed before the value of using lecithin in treating Alzheimers patients can be confirmed, but it is an inexpensive, harmless, and readily available supplement.

Lecitihin is most commonly derived from soy, a food that has suffered from significant genetic modification in recent years. Unless lecithin is obtained from sources that are guaranteed to be organic and non-GMO, it may be best to avoid this product. Even then increasing contamination from genetically modified plants raises questions of safety. Patients with known soy allergy should also avoid soy lecithin. Non soy based lecithin products are becoming more available on the market, which may be a better choice in attempting to avoid genetic modification.

Phosphotidylserine at doses of 100 mg three times a day has been shown to stabilize integrity of brain cell membranes, increase energy production in brain cells and enhance and mimic the actions of acetylcholine. Its antioxidant activity is specific to the brain cells. Folic acid, vitamin B12, and the presence of adequate essential fatty acids help the brain to produce its own phosphotidylserine.[128]

L-acetyl carnitine is important for the transport of long chain fatty acids into the mitochondria of brain cells. The mitochondria are structures that are responsible for energy production in the cell. L-acetyl carnitine occurs naturally in the brain and has a structural similarity to acetylcholine. It acts as an antioxidant within the brain cell, stabilizes cell membrane integrity and has been shown to be helpful in age-related depression, early Alzheimer's, and memory impairment.[129] The standard oral dose is 500 mg three times a day.

Antioxidants, including vitamins C, A, and E, alpha lipoic acid, co-enzyme Q-10, and selenium are all important to help address and prevent further oxidative damage to brain tissue. Needless to say an optimal diet is essential. Foods rich in flavonoids will be especially protective in reducing inflammation and oxidative stress.

Leaves harvested from the Ginkgo biloba tree are well known for their ability to improve cognitive function.[130] Ginkgo increases cerebral circulation, decreases platelet aggregation and is rich in antioxidants. It has been shown to normalize acetylcholine receptors in the area of the brain most affected by Alzheimer's (hippocampus).[131,132] Like any of these recommendations, Ginkgo is most effective in early onset Alzheimer's. It should be considered in early dementia, and in symptoms resulting from vascular insufficiency due to carotid artery occlusion.

Standardized extracts of 24% ginkgo flavoglycosides are often used in studies. Doses recommended are 80 mg three times a day. I do not personally find that standardized extracts are necessary. Clinical experience suggests that 60 drops of tincture taken three times a day may be employed with equally good results.

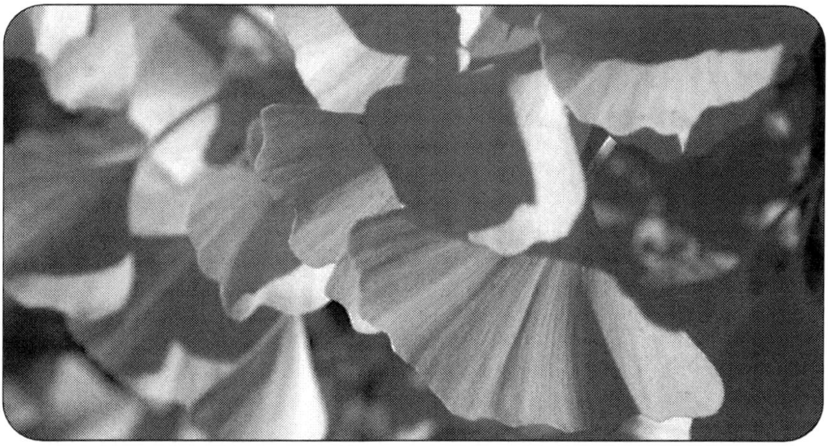

Ginkgo *Photo courtesy of Orna Izakson N.D.*

Vinca minor also increases circulation to the cerebral cortex.[133] Clinically, Vinca seems to be powerfully synergistic when combined with ginkgo, where flavonoids and increased circulation to the brain may help prevent and reverse ischemic damage. Other actions of Vinca include an ability to decrease peripheral resistance in blood vessels, making it useful as an antihypertensive. Like Crataegus, it is a coronary vessel vasodilator where it may be useful in the treatment of angina. Vinca minor contains some of the same anti-neoplastic constituents as Catharanthus rosea and may be considered as part of a treatment plan for patients struggling with cancer.[134]

While Vinca minor certainly appears to be neuroprotective and neuroregenerative, there are also some suggestions that it may be protective to other tissues as well. For the eyes it can aid in improving night vision and preventing or slowing macular degeneration.[135]

Vinca minor is also hemostatic and astringent. Constituents include tannins, glucides, flavonoids, and multiple alkaloids, including vincristine and vincamine.

A related plant, Vinca major, which is also astringent, does not appear to have the ability to increase cerebral blood flow.

Doses of 6 drops three times a day in formula are quite effective. Overdose can result in a serious, even life threatening drop in blood pressure.

Rosemary has a long standing reputation in the treatment of memory loss and decreased mental alertness. As is the case with so many "old wives tales," the familiar expression "Rosemary for Remembrance" has merit. Constituents include choline as well as essential oils and resins. It has antioxidant, nervine, and antidepressant actions as well as being a chloretic and cholagogue, stimulating a sluggish gall bladder back to normal function. Herbalist Maude Grieve tells us rosemary strengthens the brain, soothes the nerves, and may prove helpful for functional heart palpitations.

Traditionally associated with fidelity, rosemary was considered especially protective to lovers. A wreath of rosemary might be worn by the bride in wedding ceremonies. Other uses include treatment of hypercholesterolemia, tinnitus, migraines, and Meniere's disease.

A 1:5 extract of rosemary tincture may be dosed at 10-30 drops up to four times a day.

Bacopa monniera, a nervine from India, has been shown to improve memory, mental alertness, ability to focus, and retention in learning. Bacopa may be considered for the patient recovering from stroke as well as in treatment of cognitive disorders.

Centella asiatica (gotu kola) is deeply healing and rejuvenative to the nervous system and brain, where it enhances cognitive abilities and increases memory. It is calming and adaptogenic. Ayurvedic physician, Dr. Vasant Lad tells us that gotu kola is one of the most important rejuvenating herbs for the brain and nervous system in Ayurvedic medicine.

Gotu kola is also indicated as a blood cleanser in skin diseases, and as an immune tonic. This latter action may be due to adaptogenic properties. Recent research suggests the plant may be useful in encouraging healthy connective tissue repair, especially in patients who are prone to keloid formation or excessive scar tissue.[136]

Because this plant is rich in minerals and mild in taste, I prefer to give it as a powder in doses of 1/2 to 1 teaspoon 1 - 4 times per day. The tea is delicious and may be dosed at one tablespoon per cup, taken 2 - 4 cups per day. Tincture of a 1:1 extract may be dispensed at up to 60 drops four times daily.

Crataegus spp (hawthorne), another plant rich in flavonoids and antioxidants, strengthens, nourishes, and protects the heart and blood vessels. It is especially indicated where cardiovascular deficits may be playing a part in cognitive decline, but it should be considered as a base for any patient with cognitive impairment. (See chapter on hawthorne for more.)

Homeopathy has shown itself to be a powerful ally in treating cognitive dysfunction. Homeopathic Pulsatilla may be useful when patients exhibit teariness and grief at loss of mental capabilities. Baryta caronicum may be appropriate when the patient is clingy and childlike whereas Anacardium will be more indicated when belligerence accompanies declining mental function.

One man who developed a tendency to rages as his cognitive function declined did well with homeopathic Anacardium. The increasing belligerence and paranoia that accompanied episodes of confusion were a complete change in personality for this man and were hugely ameliorated by the remedy.

Other homeopathic remedies should also be considered as indicated by the patient's presentation.

Elderly patients with minimal symptoms of cognitive decline may suddenly exhibit complete disorientation with an acute disease or when unexpected changes arise. Any patient who experiences a sudden decline in cognition should be medically evaluated to rule out impending stroke, or metabolic disturbances. A urinalysis is warranted at the outset in any elderly patient with sudden change in mental state, as occult urinary tract infections can manifest with sudden confusion as the only presenting symptom in elders.

One patient experienced a significant decline in mental function when she was moved from her home to another state to be closer to family. Another woman, who was doing well on herbs, regular injections of vitamin B12, and an LM potency of Pulsatilla, became agitated and completely disoriented during an episode of flu. She quickly responded to Pulsatilla 200C dosed every 4 hours, which cleared up her cough and flu as well.

Actinic Keratosis and Sun Damaged Skin

Herbal medicine lends itself well to the treatment of precancerous conditions of the skin. Three herbs that have served well in my practice for treating these lesions are Larrea spp. (Chaparral), Sanguinaria canadensis (Bloodroot), and Croton spp. (Dragon's Blood).

Chapparal (Larrea tridentata/Larrea divaricata)
Zygophyllaceae

Leaves, twigs, seeds and flowers of chaparral have tradionally been prepared as a tea. Leaves have historically been either infused or decocted. The plant has a very strong taste and one pinch of herb per cup of water will often provide sufficient medicine without overly offending the taste buds. I personally find the tea to be preferable, because chaparral seems to let us know, by our response to the taste, whether it is the appropriate medicine for us in that moment. Doses vary in the literature however, going up to as much as 1 tablespoon of infused leaves and twigs per pint of water. Another writer suggests preparing the herb as a decoction using a handful of leaves per 1 - 2 pints of water, while still other sources suggest as much as 1 tablespoon per cup of water infused for 25 minutes. However, due to controversy about possible hepatotoxicity with internal dosing of this plant, lower doses may be preferable. Topical applications appear to be totally safe.

Despite long standing historical use of chaparral as a tea, combined with the fact that some of the most medically significant constituents are more soluble in water than alcohol, the tincture does appear to be effective in clinical practice, although tea may be the safer and more effective route of administration. While tincture may be dosed at 10 - 60 drops 1 - 4 times daily, I have never gone over 15 drops twice a day. Some herbalists feel that the more modern use of tincture may be creating problems and suggest that traditional use of tea may be safer.

The desert chaparral, also known as creosote bush and grease wood, is a strong, very distinctive smelling bush with small, opposite, bifolate green to yellow-green resinous leaves. Five-petaled yellow flowers bloom in spring or after a rain and are attractive to a wide variety of bees. Fruits are small and have a white furry coat. In order to preserve water and survive the harsh desert climate, Chaparral puts out a growth inhibitory substance that prevents other plants from germinating in the soil nearby, including the sprouts of its own seeds. Sections of stem near the leaves have the ability to photosynthesize.

The leaves contain one of the strongest known anti-oxidants, nordihydroguaiaretic acid (NDGA). This constituent has been shown to have anti-cancer, anti-inflammatory, and anti-bacterial properties. (Brinker) The many flavonoids present in the plant enhance NDGA's anti-inflammatory and anti-oxidant properties, inhibit platelet aggregation and add anti-viral, anti-fungal, and anti-allergic properties.

Asthmatic patients may obtain relief from chaparral due to its activity as a lipoxygenase inhibitor, and its ability to block the release of histamine, prostaglandins, and SRS-A (slow reacting substance of anaphylaxis.) The plant is also an expectorant.

Chaparral leaves have been used for a wide variety of complaints including arthritis, asthma, allergy, autoimmune disease, respiratory infection, genito-urinary symptoms, menstrual cramps, neuritis, diarrhea, and a variety of skin conditions. Despite modern concerns over potential hepatotoxicity with internal dosing, chaparral can also be a helpful aid in enhancing liver and digestive function.

Chaparral has a folk reputation for being efficacious in the treatment of cancer. Certainly the significant anti-oxidant activity generated by its high flavonoid content and the presence of NDGA would substantiate such claims. In fact, NDGA has been found to be inhibitory to both aerobic and anaerobic glycolysis in cancer cells, thereby diminishing the ability of these cells to produce energy.[137] In addition, NDGA has been shown to block the mutagenicity of some carcinogenic substances, and inhibit induction of biochemical pathways that might otherwise encourage tumor growth.[138] However, the results of modern research are contradictory. Humans and animal trials showed very little result when either chaparral tea or NDGA were administered for the treatment of cancer. Some patients even seemed to experience an increase in tumor growth.[139] Despite impressive evidence that chaparral is cytotoxic to cancer cells and inhibitory to tumor growth,[140] scientific evidence that chaparral is indeed an effective agent in the treatment of cancer remains controversial.

The late Dr. Bill Mitchell, naturopathic physician, herbalist, and cofounder of Bastyr University, once told a story of a woman who came to his clinic in very late stages of cancer. She never followed up after the first visit, and he presumed she had simply passed away soon thereafter. A year later he happened to see her in a public setting, looking robust and healthy. Surprised to find her appearing so vital, he approached her and asked what she had done to help herself. Her response … "I drank huge quantities of chaparral tea."

There are many isolated tales of chaparral curing folks of their cancer. While it does not bode well to ignore or underestimate the validity of these stories, at the same time it also behooves us to acknowledge the puzzling contradictions in both scientific and clinical evidence. Needless to say, self treatment of serious conditions like cancer is not recommended.

In clinical practice, chaparral has proven very useful in reducing precancerous lesions on the skin, particularly the brown spots of sun-damaged skin (actinic keratoses). It is important to be persistent with topical application if the treatment is to be effective and nightly application is advised. Internal use of tincture, 15 drops twice daily or a daily cup or two of tea, (the preferred route of admistration) aids to increase the speed and efficacy of treatment.

Reports that ingestion of chaparral may be linked to hepatotoxicity are as controversial as the use of chaparral in the treatment of cancer. Some herbalists feel that the more modern tinctured preparation of the herb may result in concentration of potentially hepatotoxic constituents not present in a water extract. Others are of the opinion that the encapsulated herb offers increased potential for overdose, and should, therefore, be avoided. In one study that did demonstrate potential hepatotoxicity NDGA was administered intra-peritoneally to mice,[141] probably not the most likely route of ingestion for your average herb consumer. Retrospective studies do exist that connect the ingestion of chaparral (in humans) with significant hepato and nephrotoxicity.[142] Other reports demonstrate the safety of chaparral in low doses used in the clinical setting.[143]

Amidst all these contradictions, chaparral can only be admired for its mysterious ability to resist reductionistic dissection. Perhaps part of its medicine is to restore some humility to the human race, if such a feat is indeed possible.

Below are a few quotes from students who have shared this plant in class and sat with its medicine for a time:

> *"It settled my stomach after the large meal we just finished."*
>
> *"Good for digestion."*
>
> *"Cooling."*
>
> *"Refreshing, cleansing, then a pungent taste and it took my attention to my core. (abdomen)"*
>
> *"Strong cleanser. Draws out poisons."*
>
> *"Smells and tastes like a hospital, anti-septic."*
>
> *"Astringent, bitter, chewy, sticks to my teeth."*
>
> *"Strong!"*

"You cannot rush into this medicine."
"You need to work with the plant."
"Not a plant for everyone."
"Strong, but I don't feel like it would harm me."
"Safe, peaceful, calming."
"Memories of home."

Immediately after my first personal experience with ingestion of chaparral, I developed an uncontrollable urge to clean the office and later my home. The obsession to clean was so strong that my receptionist remarked at my unusual behavior. I am not generally untidy, but neither am I ever as assiduous in my need to clean as I was that day!

Legend tells us that chaparral will call out and draw you to it. I didn't hear that legend until some years after chaparral called me to the Southwest. It was mid-autumn, when I began to experience an overwhelming need to lie down under a chaparral bush, a plant I had never actually met in person, residing as I do in the wet rainy Pacific Northwest. The intensely strong craving persisted over some weeks and I was rather at a loss for what to do about it, when I received a phone call from the organizers of the Southwest Conference on Botanical Medicine inviting me to speak that spring. I knew the answer had to be yes!

Sanguinaria canadensis (Bloodroot)

Sanguinaria is one of the main ingredients in the "Black Salve" used by some practitioners as a topical agent in the treatment of cancer, where it is reputed to draw cancer from the body. When the salve is applied topically it creates an ulcer that can become quite large and painful. One patient who was being treated for breast cancer by another physician developed a wound that covered half the affected breast and was easily as tender and painful as it was disfiguring. One wonders if conventional surgery would not have been kinder.

Most reasonable practitioners do not recommend the use of black salve for internal cancers, partly because it is so disfiguring and painful and its efficacy in highly debated.

Although the use of the salve is controversial, it can be considered for skin cancers. I have found it to be successful for treating basal cell carcinomas of the skin and another physician reported to me that her older brother was able to clear up a squamous cell carcinoma on his face using black salve.

Some practitioners report success using black salve in the topical treatment of malignant melanoma.

These conditions should all be treated with the supervision of a qualified health care practitioner.

As there are a few salves on the market labelel "black salve," it is important to note that the black salve utilized for cancer must contain both Sanguinaria and zinc chloride, if it is to be used successfully. I do not recommend using black salve for cancers, other than skin cancer, and no one should be self-treating any cancer without medical supervision.

The salve can also be considered when simpler methods do not remove precancerous lesions like actinic keratoses, or actinic lentigo (brown sun spots that are associated with aging). These latter conditions usually respond to topical applications of chaparral (Larrea tridentata), Sanguinaria alone or the two herbs in combination. However, unless you are a qualified health care practitioner, please do not attempt to treat cancer of any sort on your own.

Sanguinaria is used topically as part of an "escharotic treatment" for advanced cervical dysplasias (abnormal precancerous cells found on routine pap smears). While there seems to be a movement within the naturopathic profession toward more aggressive surgical debridement of abnormal cells in these cases, many of us still rely on these traditional methods which have held us in good stead over the years. Unlike the surgical LEEP procedure, the escharotic treatment does not carry the risk of scarring the endocervical canal.

Dr. Bill Mitchell reported success applying 3 drops of the tincture topically to the cervix in cases of cervical erosion.

Sanguinaria's anti-fungal properties make it a consideration for topical treatment of fungal infections on the skin, such as tinea (ringworm). Such topical treatment should always be accompanied by internal support of the immune system. A tincture of equal parts of the anti-fungal herbs Spilanthes and Usnea taken internally can be dosed at 60 drops 3 times a day for optimal benefit.

Sanguinaria is also anti-viral, and as mentioned earlier, a powder of Sanguinaria wetted down with a drop or so of the essential oil of Thuja plicata will remove the most stubborn of warts. It may be applied to the venereal warts of HPV as well. When it is difficult to obtain powdered herb a tincture of Sanguinaria mixed with the Thuja essntial oil will also work, although not as quickly. Effects are enhanced when an anti-viral formula of herbs is taken internally.

The plant is also anti-inflammatory and anti-bacterial. Ten drops of the tincture mixed with a tablespoon or two of water makes a useful mouthwash helping to decrease plaque and inhibit bacterial growth. Like most other mouthwashes, the Sanguinaria mixture should not be swallowed as the plant does have potential toxicity.

Sanguinaria taken internally can be highly toxic if proper dosing is not followed and those doses are very low. Most sources recommend using 1 - 2 drops of a 1:1.1 fresh plant tincture 1 - 4 times per day in acute conditions, dropping to 1 - 2 drops daily for chronic ongoing symptoms. Maximum dosing for more acute conditions should not exceed 1 - 2 drops every 2 - 4 hours while awake. These drop doses are usually taken diluted in water.

Sanguinaria has most often been used as an expectorant, where it is specifically indicated when the patient complains of burning, itching, irritation or tickling in the mucous membranes of the respiratory tract with a sense of constriction in the throat or in the chest behind the sternum. Expectoration may be profuse or difficult and scanty, with Sanguinaria acting to normalize secretions in either case. Discharges may be thin and acrid, and pains, if present, will be described as sharp and lancinating. Sanguinaria will act as an effective anti-spasmodic when used internally, making it useful for spasmodic coughs and dyspnea. The plant is useful after bronchitis or pneumonia where a chronic cough persists and the patient is debilitated.

In cases where sore throat with burning and irritation accompany the symptom picture, 1 - 2 drops of the tincture can be mixed in a tablespoon of water and gargled, then swallowed or spit into the sink. If the herb is swallowed it is important to follow dosing closely. Mucous membranes of the pharynx will be red and inflamed on examination when Sanguinaria is indicated.

The patient who responds well to the internal dosing of Sanguinaria may be chilly with cold hands and feet.

An excellent alterative, Sanguinaria stimulates the liver and acts as a mild cholagogue, diaphoretic, and diuretic. It has been used to treat sick, congestive headache due to biliary stasis, with 1 - 2 drop doses being administered every 2 - 3 hours as needed.

The root and rhizome are most commonly used, although other sources report use of the whole plant.

Constituents include multiple isoquinoline alkaloids including sanguinarine, sanguidaridine, sanguidimerine, sanguirubine, sanguilutine, oxysanguidarine, chelerythrine, gamma homo-chelidonine, berberine, captisine, chelilutine, protopine, alpha & beta allocrytopine and others. Of particular interest is the berberine, also present in Hydrastis Canadensis (goldenseal), and Mahonia spp. (Oregon grape root). Berberine is reputed to contribute significantly to the anti-microbial activity of these plants. Sanguinarine & chelerythrine are also found in Chelidonium majus (greater celandine).

I have personally only used this herb for topical applications. The herb is not abundant in nature and should therefore be used judiciously.

Dragon's Blood (Croton spp.) Euphobiaceae

After discovering that this potent Amazonian rain forest herb is high in antioxidant flavonoids, I began adding it to my protocol for the topical treatment of precancerous skin lesions. The deep reddish color of the plant tincture reflects the high flavonoid content.

Because Chapparal is so prolific on the desert, it is probably a better first choice then importing an herb from the rain forest. However, if lesions are stubborn and unresponsive, dragon's blood can be a good alternative. Like chapparal and blood root, the tincture is applied at bedtime and left on the skin overnight. Care should be taken, as it will easily stain clothing.

The medicine is gathered from the sap of the Croton lechleri or Croton salutaris tree, which seeps out of cut bark like blood from a wound. It has been used traditionally to staunch hemorrhage and as a protective covering for wounds.

Internally, it is anti-viral, where it may be considered for herpes infections, HIV, and hepatitis, as well as seasonal influenza. Antibacterial and antifungal activities other properties credited to this herb. It has anti-inflammatory as well as wound healing properties where it has proven itself effective in healing ulcers of the mouth and gastrointestinal tract. Dragon's blood has also been shown to be useful in the treatment of cancer,[144] perhaps at least in part due to its high flavonoid content. It is used both internally and externally for hemorrhage. Recent research validates its folk use as a vulnerary.[145]

The long list of constituents includes several alkaloids, flavonoids, phenols, phytosterols, diterpenes, and lignans. The presence of catechins suggests it may have hepatoprotective qualities.

Recommended dose is 10 - 25 drops 3 times per day. I know of no contraindications for this plant, except perhaps pregnancy. In my practice I have so far only used this herb externally.

Cataracts

Cataracts, formed by an opacity that occurs in the lens of the eye, are primarily found in people over the age of 60. As they tend to develop gradually, cataracts may go unnoticed until picked up on a routine eye exam. When symptoms are present there may be cloudy vision, decreased night vision, increased sensitivity to light, or double vision occurring only in one eye. Lights may appear to be surrounded by a halo.

If caught early, cataracts respond well to an herbal preparation of Cineraria maritima placed into the affected eye(s). Various products are available on the market and dosage should be in keeping with recommendations for the specific product being used.

Internal use of lutein, bilberry, and an abundance of antioxidant/anthocyanin rich foods such as blueberries, blackberries, cherries, and pomegranates should also be included in the treatment protocol.

Gout

Acute gouty arthritis classically presents with inflammation, redness, and swelling involving only one joint. The disease most commonly affects the base of the great toe, but symptoms can occur in other joints with feet, ankles, knees, hands, and wrists all being potential sites for inflammation. Affected areas are often exquisitely tender and sensitive to the slightest touch. The condition can become chronic, manifesting as recurrent episodes over time.

Gout is caused by an accumulation of uric acid in the blood stream which crystalizes and gets deposited in the joint. Blood tests may or may not reveal an elevation of uric acid in the serum, even with an acute presentation, but if uric acid is increased the diagnosis is more certain. Elevations in uric acid in the absence of symptoms suggest a vulnerability to developing gout or uric acid kidney stones.

Because uric acid is excreted through the kidneys, keeping up a good intake of fluids is essential in managing acute cases of gout and preventing kidney stones or further episodes of arthritic symptoms.

When treating gout, the diet should be low in purine rich foods. Sardines, lobster, shrimp, herring, anchovies, organ meats, high fructose corn syrup, and alcohol have all been linked to flare ups of gouty arthritis. All meats, fish, and poultry contain purines and these foods should be kept minimal in the diet.

If tolerated, a few days of only fresh vegetables and anthocyanin-rich berries may be used as a short term therapeutic intervention during acute flare-ups. Cherries have long been used in the treatment of gout. Several ounces of cherry juice, 1 cup of frozen dark cherries, or 1/2 cup of dried cherries per day can help reduce inflammation in acute gout and regular daily ingestion may aid in preventing recurrence. While blueberries, strawberries, blackberries and pomegranates also contain anthocyanins, cherries have been the historical remedy for gout.

Nettles, couch grass, juniper berries, and pipsissewa have all been used in the management of gout and these urinary tract tonics are probably acting at least in part by enhancing urinary excretion of uric acid. Juniper also works by preventing crystallization of uric acid while flavonoids present in the ripe berries lend anti-inflammatory and anti-oxidant activity.

Although the herb Colchicum autumnale (autumn crocus) has been used for the treatment of gout throughout the ages, the herb is highly toxic and I have not seen enough results with its use to warrant recommending it. Should you choose to work with it mix 10 drops of the herb in 4 ounces of water and dispense 1 teaspoon every 1 to 4 hours. Maximum dose over a week's time should be no greater than 5 ml. although some practitioners have used double that dose in acute cases. The alkaloid colchicine is considered to be the active ingredient as well as the source of toxicity.

Symptoms of toxicity with Colchicum affect the gastrointestinal tract beginning with nausea and vomiting which can then progress to violent spasmodic purging, bloody diarrhea, hypovolemic shock, and collapse. One patient who was struggling with resistant symptoms of gout did develop some nausea which resolved when he lowered the dose. Although I have no compunctions about using this herb, I personally find that the homeopathic version is far more effective and a whole lot safer.

Homeopathic Colchicum 30C given four times per day has proven highly effective at diminishing symptoms of acute gout in fairly short order. Toxicity is nonexistent with the homeopathic preparation.

Juniperus communis (Juniper) Cupressaceae

Juniper is best employed as a tonic to enhance liver, kidney, and digestive function. The ripe berries, which are actually cones, contain bitters that stimulate the liver and digestive tract. They are also full of essential oils including thujone, limonene, camphor, alpha and beta pinene, myrcene, terpinene, and borneol among others. These essential oils add carminative activity that helps prevent eructations, flatulence, and indigestion. Juniper has significant diuretic properties and has historically been employed for reducing the swelling and fluid retention of "dropsy" or what we now call congestive heart failure. Flavones provide anti-inflammatory and anti-oxidant properties.

The hydropath and herbalist Father Kneipp (1821-1897) noticed that when he had patients take juniper berries to enhance kidney and digestive function before initiating hydrotherapy, the water treatments were better tolerated and more beneficial. Father Kneipp had his patients chew 5 berries on day one, adding a berry each day until the patient was ingesting 30 berries a day. The patient then reversed the process such that they ate 29 berries the next day, 28 berries the day after and so on until they were back to the original 5 berries.[146] Every self-respecting herbalist should take the opportunity to taste juniper berries to fully appreciate Father Kneipp's prescription. The sweet berry flavor combines with bitters and abundant essential oils to create a very strong taste.

Juniper is often used in formulas for acute urinary cystitis when infection is confined to the bladder and not progressing into pyelonephritis (kidney infection). The large number of essential oils in the berries contributes significant anti-microbial actions in the urinary tract, but juniper should be avoided in the presence of active inflammation in the kidneys.

Leaves and berries of juniper have been used for spiritual protection by many cultures, where they may be ingested, worn on the body, placed over doorways, or burned as a smudge. Physicians and herbalists of the past often chewed juniper berries as they went about their rounds during epidemic illnesses to avoid getting ill.

One of the spiritual gifts of juniper is discernment and I often carry a few berries with me or burn the leaves as a smudge when I find the need for a little help in that area. The ripe berries of juniper are harvested after being on the tree or bush for a year, but the harvester must differentiate these mostly purple blue ripe berries that are still a bit green from the mostly green unripe berries that are slightly blue. The medicine of discernment is further illustrated if we think of the kidneys as an organ of discrimination in their role of deciding which substances are to be retained and which are to be excreted. Finally the issue of discernment comes up again when we prescribe, as we must be most assiduous in differentiating simple bladder symptoms from inflammation in the kidneys.

The twisted rugged trunks, tested by fierce mountain or desert winter winds, suggest that a stubborn strength may be imparted to the wearer who feels the need for some extra stamina and support.

The leaves of juniper make a sweet cleansing smudge that has come to be one of my favorites for use in prayer and ceremony.

A reasonable dose of Juniper is 5 - 20 drops three times per day. It combines well with other urinary and digestive tonics. The herb should be ingested before meals to enhance its digestive stimulating properties. A few berries can be chewed each day or a tea may be made by infusing as much as one teaspoon of ripe berries per cup and taking one cup before each meal.

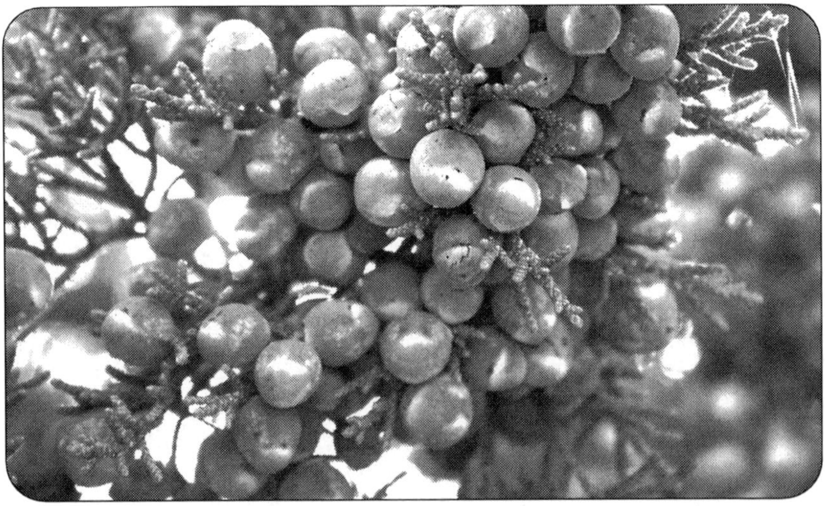

Juniper Berries *Photo courtesy of MacKenzie Duffy*

Most sources advise against taking juniper internally for more than four to six weeks at one time.

Conventional herbal wisdom recommends against using juni-per if there is any indication of kidney disease, as it is thought that the stimulating essential oils are likely to aggravate an already compromised kidney. While doing some research recently, I happened to come across the website of an herbal-ist practicing in New Zealand who claims to have uncovered information disputing this assertion. (Richard Whelan, Medical Herbalist, M.H. MNZAMH http://www.rjwhelan.co.nz/herbs February 2014.) After checking a few of the old books I discovered that King's American Dispensary, a hallowed and most reliable text from the Eclectics, actually recommends the use of juniper for "pyelitis, pyelo-nephritis, and cystitis when chronic." [147] (Whalen also places this quote on his website.) The Eclectic physician Felter[148] tells us juniper is indicated for "uncomplicated renal hyperaemia or congestion... if albumen is present... chronic nephritis, chronic pyelitis... and after acute nephritis."

Felter does warn against its use if there is active fever or inflammation in the kidneys which strongly suggests that juniper should still be assiduously avoided in acute pyelonephritis. Physiomedicalist Dr. William Cook concurs when he warns against the use of juniper in inflammatory conditions.[149]

Maud Grieve appears to recommend the essential oil in kidney conditions when she writes "Oil of Juniper is given as a diuretic, stomachic, and carminative in indigestion, flatulence, and diseases of the kidney and bladder." [150]

Further research uncovered an article in Medical Herbalism written by the very reputable herbalist and researcher Kerry Bone [151] who shared results reported at the 24th International Symposium on Essential Oils in Berlin. Presenters who had done a literature review on juniper from 1844 through 1993 seemed to agree that the toxicity of the essential oils to the kidney has been largely overstated, concluding that ripe juniper berries were unlikely to cause renal damage when used in therapeutic doses. Their literature review revealed a report of animal fatalities resulting from ingestion of juniper oils with high levels of alpha and beta pinene, two essential oils known to be irritating to renal tissue. It is suspected that this report is responsible for the current view of juniper as a kidney irritant. A subsequent, more recent study done on rats with large doses of oils not so high in the offending pinenes revealed no renal irritation when ingested.[152]

Alpha and beta pinene are higher in unripe berries, needles, and branches, suggesting that the essential oils that caused the animal fatalities may have been contaminated with unripe berries or plant parts not appropriate for ingestion[153]. Paul Bergner, herbalist, lecturer, and editor of Medical Herbalism, substantiates the importance of using only ripe berries when he writes that the 1947 US Dispensary says the essential oils of juniper berries are changed into resins as the berries ripen.[154]

Reliable sources of juniper are absolutely imperative to avoid contamination with plant parts that are more concentrated in the problematic essential oils. If the manufacture of essential oils includes these contaminants, and not just ripe berries, the possibility of kidney irritation may be increased.

While the writings of the Eclectics suggest we may be overly cautious in avoiding juniper in the treatment of renal disease, there are a whole host of other herbs to use in active kidney disease that are less controversial and probably a whole lot safer.

I still prefer to use the whole berry, avoiding the internal use of the essential oil, and continue to reserve its use primarily as a kidney and digestive tonic and alterative. I believe Paul Bergner concurs when he writes that juniper berries "are more appropriate in conditions of deficiency and laxity of the tissues than in conditions of excess or inflammation." [155]

(For more information on herbal treatments for renal pathologies see the work of Sharol Tilgner N.D. "The Contented Kidney" www.herbaltransitions.com/Kidney%20Health.pdf and the work of Eric Yarnell N.D.)

Chapter 21
Appendicitis

Appendicitis

As we approach printing and the book is all laid out by my graphic designer, I realize that this little tidbit was left out of the chapter on digestion. While I could leave it out altogether, I chose instead to tack it on at the end.

Acute appendicitis occurs as a result of an inflammatory response to bacterial invasion of the wall of the appendix, the small tube like sac that extends from the cecum. If the situation becomes serious enough the appendix may rupture, spreading bacteria into the abdominal cavity and causing peritonitis. However, the appendix may also heal on its own or if it does rupture, infected material may remain confined near the appendix and not result in a full blown case of peritonitis. While appendicitis can be managed conservatively in early stages, peritonitis is a such serious life threatening condition that any suspicion of appendicitis should not be treated lightly.

Appendicitis usually starts out as abdominal pain that is felt diffusely throughout abdomen. There may be nausea, vomiting, and loss of appetite. The patient will initially be unable to pinpoint an exact location of the pain and early symptoms can easily be mistaken for a case of gastroenteritis. I often find myself assuring people who complain that their doctor did not pick up a diagnosis of appendicitis at the outset, that it can be an easy condition to miss until symptoms progress.

When pain does localize, it will typically focus in the right lower quadrant of the abdomen, midway between the umbilicus and the anterior aspect of the ileac crest (hip bone). This area is called McBurney's point and is specific for a diagnosis of appendicitis. There may be rebound tenderness once peritoneal irritation has set in. Rebound tenderness is pain that is worse when the physician quickly removes his or her hand after palpating the tender area of the abdomen.

Blood work will reveal an elevated white blood count (WBC) but again this may be normal or only slightly elevated in early stages of the disease. Imaging utilizing X-rays, ultrasound, or computerized tomography (CT scan) may help confirm the diagnosis.

Most cases of appendicitis will respond to one of a few homeopathic remedies.

If symptoms of abdominal pain come on suddenly, homeopathic Belladonna should be considered. Pains indicating the use of Belladonna are likely to be intense and throbbing.

Bryonia symptoms will be slower in onset, but pain will be worse with even the slightest motion. As with Belladonna, pains may be intense, but onset will be gradual and the quality of the pain is likely to be more of a sharp stitching character.

Iris tenax is the remedy to consider when Bryonia and Belladonna do not seem indicated.

In cases where symptoms are severe or progressing rapidly, the remedy may be given as the patient heads to the emergency room. Sometimes by the time the patient arrives at the hospital the remedy has begun to act and symptoms may already be abating enough to allow for conservative monitoring and avoidance of surgery.

I have had occasion to use both Bryonia and Iris tenax in the treatment of appendicitis with excellent results.

Footnotes

Chapter 3

[1] Lee CH, Kim JM, Kim DH, Park SJ, Liu X, Cai M, Hong JG, Park JH, Ryu JH, *"Effects of Sun Ginseng on Memory Enhancement and Hippocampal Neurogenesis,"* Phytother Res. 2012 Oct 29. doi: 10.1002/ptr.4873.

[2] Il Woo Joo, Jae Hwan Ryu, Han Jin Oh, *"The Influence of Sam-Chil-Geun (Panax Notoginseng) on the Serum Lipid Levels and Inflammations of Rats with Hyperlipidemia Induced by Poloxamer-407,"* Yonsei Med J. 2010 July 1; 51(4): 504-510.

[3] Doa'a A Ibrahim, *"Study of the Effect of Panax Ginseng versus Gliclazide on Hyperglycaemia Induced by Dexamethasone in Experimental Animals,"* Sultan Qaboos Univ Med J. 2009 April; 9(1): 63-69.

[4] Hobbs, Christopher, L.Ac., Goldberg, Alicia, Mcguffin, Michael, Upton, Roy, Botanical Safety Handbook, American Herbal Products Association, CRC Press LLC., Boca Taton, Fla, 1997

[5] Cicero, AF, et. al., *Effects of Siberian ginseng (Eleutherococcus senticocsus maxim.) on elderly quality of life: a randomized trial.*, Arch Gerontol Geriatri Suppl, 2004; (9): 69-73

[6] Panda S, Kar A, Changes in thyroid hormone concentrations after administration of ashwaghanda root extract to adult male mice., J Pharm Phamacol 1998 Sep; 50 (9): 1065- 8

[7] Ibid.

[8] Reis SR, Valente LM, Sampaio AL, Siani AC, Gandini M, Azeredo EL, D'Avila LA, Mazzei JL, Henriques MG, Kubelka CF. *"Immunomodulating and antiviral activities of Uncaria tomentosa on human monocytes infected with Dengue Virus-2."* Int Immunopharmacol. 2008 Mar;8(3):468-76. Epub 2007 Dec 26.

[9] Pilarski R, Filip B, Wietrzyk J, Kura_ M, Gulewicz K., Phytomedicine. *"Anticancer activity of the Uncaria tomentosa (Willd.) DC. preparations with different oxindole alkaloid composition,"* 2010 Dec 1;17(14):1133-9. Epub 2010 Jun 25.

[10] Sasaki S, et al, "*Studies on the mechanism of action of asiaticoside (Madecassol) on experimental granulation tissue and cultured fibroblasts and its clinical application in systemic scleroderma,*" Acta Diabetologica Latina 52: 141 - 50, 1972.

[11] Ming ZJ, Liu SZ, Cao L., "*Effect of total glucosides of Centella asiatica on antagonizing liver fibrosis induced by dimethylnitrosamine in rats,*" Zhongguo Zhong Xi Yi Jie He Za Zhi. , "2004 Aug;24(8):731- 4 [Article in Chinese]

[12] Singh S, Taneja M, Majumdar DK, "*Biological activities of Ocimum sanctum L. fixed oil--an overview,*" Indian J Exp Biol. 2007 May;45(5):403-12.

[13] Prasad S, Yadav VR, Kannappan R, Aggarwal BB, "*Ursolic acid, a pentacyclin triterpene, potentiates TRAIL-induced apoptosis through p53-independent up-regulation of death receptors: evidence for the role of reactive oxygen species and JNK.,*" J Biol Chem. 2011 Feb 18;286(7):5546-57.

[14] Lahon K, Das S., "*Hepatoprotective activity of Ocimum sanctum alcoholic leaf extract against paracetamol-induced liver damage in Albino rats.,*" Pharmacognosy Res. 2011 Jan;3(1):13-8.

[15] Agrawal P, Rai V, Singh RB, "*Randomized placebo-controlled, single blind trial of holy basil leaves in patients with noninsulin-dependent diabetes mellitus.,*" Int J Clin Pharmacol Ther. 1996 Sep;34(9):406-9.

[16] Singh S, Majumdar DK, "*Evaluation of the gastric anti-ulcer activity of fixed oil of Ocimum sanctum (Holy Basil),*" J Ethnopharmacol, 1999 April; 65(1); 13-9.

[17] Gupta P, "*Constituents of Ocimum sanctum with anti-stress activity,*" J Nat Prod, 2007 Sept; 70 (9): 1410-6.

[18] Zamansoltani F, Nassiri-Asl M, Sarookhani MR, Jahani-Hashemi H Zangivand AA, "*Antiandrogenic activities of Glycyrrhiza glabra in male rats,*" Int J Androl. 2009 Aug;32 (4):417-22.

[19] Clement C, et al., "*Effect of Maca supplementation on bovine sperm quantity and quality followed over two spermatogenic cycles,*" Theriogenology, 2010 May 7.

[20] Sanodiya BS, Thakur GS, Baghel RK, Prasad GB, Bisen PS. "*Ganoderma lucidum: a potent pharmacological macrofungus,*" Curr Pharm Biotechnol. 2009 Dec;10(8):717-42.

[21] Jan RH, Lin TY, Hsu YC, Lee SS, Lo SY, Chang M, Chen LK, Lin YL., *"Immuno-modulatory activity of Ganoderma lucidum-derived polysacharide on human monocytoid dendritic cells pulsed with Der p 1 allergen.,"* BMC Immunol. 2011 May 25;12:31.

[22] Chen WQ, Luo SH, Ll HZ, Yang H, *"Effects of ganoderma lucidum polysaccharides on serum lipids and lipoperoxidation in experimental hyperlipidemic rats,"* Zhongguo Zhong Yao Za Zhi, 2005 Sep;30(17):1358-60.[Article in Chinese]

[23] Futrakul N, Boonyen M, Patumraj S, Siriviriyakul P, Tosukhowong P, Futrakul P. *"Treatment of glomerular endothelial dysfunction in steroid-resistant nephrosis with Ganoderma lucidum, vitamins C, E and vasodilators."* Clin Hemorheol Microcirc. 2003;29(3-4):205-10.

[24] Martínez-Montemayor MM, Acevedo RR, Otero-Franqui E, Cubano LA, Dharmawardhane SF, *"Ganoderma lucidum (Reishi) inhibits cancer cell growth and expression of key molecules in inflammatory breast cancer.,"* Nutr Cancer. 2011 Oct;63(7):1085-94. Epub 2011 Sep 2.

[25] Hsieh TC, Wu JM., *"Suppression of proliferation and oxidative stress by extracts of Ganoderma lucidum in the ovarian cancer cell line OVCAR-3.,"* Int J Mol Med. 2011 Dec;28(6):1065-9. doi: 10.3892/ijmm.2011.788. Epub 2011 Sep 1.

[26] Kubo N, Myojin Y, Shimamoto F, Kashimoto N, Kyo E, Kamiya K, Watanabe H., *"Protective effects of a water-soluble extract from cultured medium of Ganoderma lucidum (Rei-shi) mycelia and Agaricus blazei murill against X-irradiation in B6C3F1 mice: Increased small intestinal crypt survival and prolongation of average time to animal death.,"* Int J Mol Med. 2005 Mar;15(3):401-6.

[27] Kim KC, Jun HJ, Kim JS, Kim IG., *"Enhancement of radiation response with combined Ganoderma lucidum and Duchesnea chrysantha extracts in human leukemia HL-60 cells.,"* Int J Mol Med . 2008 Apr;21(4):489-98.

[28] Fintelmann V, Gruenwald J., *"Efficacy and tolerability of a Rhodiola rosea extract in adults with physical and cognitive deficiencies.,"* Adv Ther. 2007 Jul-Aug;24(4):929-39.

[29] Loo WT, et. al., *"Rhodiola algida improves chemotherapy induced oral mucositis in breast cancer patients.,"* Expert Opin investing Drugs, April 2010: 19 Suppl 1: S91-100.

[30] Maslov LN, Lishmanov IuB, "*Cardioprotective and antiarrhythmic properties of Rhodiolae roseae preparation,.*" Eksp Klin Farmakol., 2007 Sep-Oct; 70(5):59-67.

[31] Ibid.

[32] Watanabe T, Watanabe M, Watanabe Y, Hotta C., "*Effects of oral administration of Pfaffia paniculata (Brazilian ginseng) on incidence of spontaneous leukemia in AKR/J mice.,*" Cancer Detect Prev. 2000;24(2):173-8.

[33] Nagamine MK, da Silva TC, Matsuzaki P, Pinello KC, Cogliati B, Pizzo CR, Akisue G, Haraguchi M, Górniak SL, Sinhorini IL, Rao KV, Barbuto JA, Dagli ML. "*Cytotoxic effects of butanolic extract from Pfaffia paniculata (Brazilian ginseng) on cultured human breast cancer cell line MCF-7 ,*" Exp Toxicol Pathol. 2009 Jan;61(1):75-82. Epub 2008 May 16.

[34] Oshima M, Gu Y., "*Pfaffia paniculata-induced changes in plasma estradiol-17beta, progesterone and testosterone levels in mice.*", J Reprod Dev. 2003 Apr;49(2):175-80.

[35] Arletti R et al, "*Stimulating property of Turnera diffusa and Pfaffia paniculata extracts on the sexual behavior of male rats.,*" Psychopharmacology (Berl), 1999 Mar, 143(1); pp. 15-9

Chapter 4

[36] Singh S, et. al., "*Antifungal activity of the alkaloids from Eschscholzia californica,*" Folia microbial (Praha), 2009; 54(3): pp. 204-6

[37] Safayhi H, et. al., "*Chamazulene: an anti-oxidant-type inhibitor of leukotriene B4 formation,*" Planta Medica; October 1994, 60(5): pp. 410-3

[38] Dorn C, et. al., "*Xanthohumol, a chalcon derived form hops, inhibits hepatic inflammation and fibrosis,*" Molec Nutri Food Res, January 2010.

[39] Dorn C. et. al., "*Xanthohumol, a prenylated chalcone derived from hops, inhibits proliferation, migration and interleukin-8 expression of hepatocellular carcinoma cells,*" Int J Oncol., February 2010; 36(2) pp. 435-41

[40] Hemachandra LP, Madhubhani P, Chandrasena R, Esala P, Chen SN, Main M, Lankin DC, Scism RA, Dietz BM, Pauli GF, Thatcher GR, Bolton JL., "*Hops (Humulus lupulus) Inhibits Oxidative Estrogen Metabolism and*

Estrogen-Induced Malignant Transformation in Human Mammary Epithelial cells (MCF-10A).," Cancer Prev Res (Phila). 2012 Jan;5(1):73-81. Epub 2011 Oct 13.

[41] Zanoli P., et. al., *"Experimental evidence of the anaphrodesiac activity of Humulus lupulus L. in naïve male rats,"* J. Ehnopharmacology, August 2009; 125(1): pp. 36 - 40

[42] Mazzanti G, Battinelli L, Pompeo C, Serrilli AM, Rossi R, Sauzullo I, Mengoni F, Vullo V., *"Inhibitory activity of Melissa officinalis L. extract on Herpes simplex virus type 2 replication.,"* Nat Prod Res. 2008;22(16):1433-40.

[43] Santini F, Vitti P, Ceccarini G, Mammoli C, Rosellini V, Pelosini C, Marsili A, Tonacchera M, Agretti P, Santoni T, Chiovato L, Pinchera A., *"In vitro assay of thyroid disruptors affecting TSH-stimulated adenylate cyclase activity.,J"* Endocrinol Invest. 2003 Oct;26(10):950-5.

[44] Auf'mkolk M, Ingbar JC, Kubota K, Amir SM, Ingbar SH, *"Extracts and auto-oxidized constituents of certain plants inhibit the receptor-binding and the biological activity of Graves' immunoglobulins."*, Endocrinology. 1985 May;116(5):1687-93.

[45] Boericke, William, M.D., Pocket Manual of Homeopathic Materia Medica, Indian Books and Periodical Syndicate, New Delhi, India

[46] The Eclectics were MDs who practiced herbal medicina in the early 1900s. They treated a wide variety of serious conditions, were very specific in their prescribing, and fortunately left a rich legacy of writings behind. Authors inclue Felter, Ellingwood, Scudder and others.

[47] Zhang Z1, Lian XY, Li S, Stringer JL.,*"Characterization of chemical ingredients and anticonvulsant activity of American skullcap (Scutellaria lateriflora).",* Phytomedicine. 2009 May;16(5):485-93. doi: 10.1016/j.phymed.2008.07.011. Epub 2008 Sep 10.

[48] Ibid.

[49] Fritz D, Venturi CR, Cargnin S, Schripsema J, Roehe PM, Montanha JA, von Poser GL., *"Herpes virus inhibitory substances from Hypericum connatum Lam., a plant used in southern Brazil to treat oral lesions."*, J Ethnopharmacol. 2007 Sep 25;113(3):517-20. Epub 2007 Jul 20.

Chapter 7

[50] Ja_arevi_ E, Williams SA, Vandas GM, Ellersieck MR, Liao C, Kannan K, Roberts RM, Geary DC, Rosenfeld CS, "*Sex and dose-dependent effects of developmental exposure to bisphenol A on anxiety and spatial learning in deer mice (Peromyscus maniculatus bairdii) offspring*," Horm Behav. 2012 Oct 7. pii: S0018-506X(12)00232-2. doi: 10.1016/j.yhbeh.2012.09.009.

[51] Parodi PW, "*Cows' milk fat components as potential anticarcinogenic agents*," J Nutr. 1997 Jun;127(6):1055-60.

[52] Kaunitz H, Dayrit CS. "*Coconut oil consumption and coronary heart disease.*," Philippine Journal of Internal Medicine, 1992;30:165-171

[53] Prior IA, Davidson F, Salmond CE, Czochanska Z. "*Cholesterol, coconuts, and diet on Polynesian atolls: a natural experiment: The Pukapuka and Tokelau Island studies*," American Journal of Clinical Nutrition, 1981;34:1552-1561

[54] Stabler SP. "*Screening the older population for cobalamin (vitamin B12) deficiency.*," J Am Geriatr Soc 1995;43:1291.

[55] Paul Bergner, "*Symphytum: Comfrey, coltsfoot, and pyrrolizidine alkaloids*," Medical Herbalism 1(1):1,3-5

[56] Cheny G, Waxler, SH, Miller IJ, "*Vitamin U therapy of peptic ulcer; experience at San Quentin Prison*," Calif Med. 1956 Jan;84(1):39-42

[57] For more detailed information I recommend the book The Seasonal Cleanse Workbook, Mind-Body Detoxifiction for the 21st Century, by Dr. Nedrow N.D., with Dr. Rod Newton D.C., available through Hidden Springs Press, Ashland, Oregon.

[58] Guyton, Arthur & Hall, Jon E., Textbook of Medical Physiology, ed.11, pp. 847 - 848

[59] Ibid.

[60] Ibid.

[61] Ruggiero Francavilla, et al., "*A Randomized Controlled Trial of Lactobacillus GG in Children With Functional Abdominal Pain*," Pediatrics, Official Journal of the American Academy of Pediatrics, 2010;126;e1445; originally published online November 15, 2010

[62] Valentina Marcone, Ettore Calzolari, Marco Bertini, *"Effectiveness of vaginal administration of Lactobacillus rhamnosus following conventional metronidazole therapy: how to lower the rate of bacterial vaginosis recurrences,"* NewMicrobiogica, 31, 429-433, 2008

Chapter 8

[63] No author listed, *"Environmental Assaults & Viral Diseases,"* Complimentary Medicine, May/June 1987, pp. 28 - 29. Although this reference is not new, it is of interest to note that this information has been available and indeed quite obvious to many, for several years.

[64] Ahmadi-Ashtiani H, Allameh A, Rastegar H, Soleimani M, Barkhordari E., *"Inhibition of cyclooxygenase-2 and inducible nitric oxide synthase by silymarin in proliferating mesenchymal stem cells: comparison with glutathione modifiers,"* J Nat Med. 2012 Jan;66(1):85-94. doi: 10.1007/s11418-011-0554-6.

Chapter 9

[65] Lee JK, Jung JS, Park SH, Park SH, Sim YB, Kim SM, Ha TS, Suh HW. *"Anti-inflammatory effect of visnagin in lipopolysaccharide-stimulated BV-2 microglial cells.,"* Arch Pharm Res. 2010 Nov;33(11):1843-50. doi: 10.1007/s12272-010-1117-1.

[66] Mitchell, William A., N.D., Plant Medicine in Practice, Using the Teachings of John Bastyr, Churchill Livingstone, Philadelphia, 1993

[67] Mitchell, William A., N.D., Plant Medicine in Practice, Using the Teachings of John Bastyr, Churchill Livingstone, Philadelphia, 1993

[68] Mitchell, William A. Jr., Plant Medicine in Practice, Using the Teachings of John Bastyr, (Philadelphia: Elsevier Science), p. 245

[69] CDC Dec 8, 2012 http://www.cdc.gov/features/pertussis/

[70] Ibid.

[71] For information on these treatments, with special indications and contraindications, please refer to Lectures in Naturopathic Hydrotherapy, by Wade Boyle N.D., and Andre Saine N.D. This book is available through the book store at the National College of Natural Medicine in Portland, OR.

[72] As of this writing I have not been able to track down the actual research but only found several references to it.

[73] Di Pierro F, Rapacioli G, Ferrara T, Togni S. "*Use of a standardized extract from Echinacea angustifolia (Polinacea) for the prevention of respiratory tract infections,*" Altern Med Rev. 2012 Mar;17(1):36-41.

[74] Hudson JB., "*Applications of the phytomedicine Echinacea purpurea (Purple Coneflower) in infectious diseases,*" J Biomed Biotechnol. 2012;2012:769896. Epub 2011 Oct 26.

[75] Mir-Rashed N, Cruz I, Jessulat M, Dumontier M, Chesnais C, Ng J, Amiguet VT, Golshani A, Arnason JT, Smith ML., "*Disruption of fungal cell wall by antifungal Echinacea extracts,*" Med Mycol. 2010 Nov;48(7):949-58.

Chapter 10

[76] Abdin, Maria, "*Possible Role for Plantago Lanceolata in the Treatment of HIV Infection?*" Townsend Letter for Doctors, June 2006, pp. 92 - 93

Chapter 11

[77] Li JX, et. al., "*Triterpenoids from Cimicifuga rhizome, a novel class of inhibitors on bone resorption and ovariectomized bone loss,*" Maturitas; 2007 Sep 20, 58 (1), pp. 59 - 69

[78] Qiu SX, et al, "*A triterpene glycoside from black cohosh that inhibits osteoclastoegensis by modulating RANKL and TNF alfa signaling pathways,*" Chem Biol; 2007 Jul 14(7), pp.

[79] Oktyabrsky O., et al, "*Assessment of anti-oxidant activity of plants using microbial test systems,*" J Applied Microbiol, 2009 Apr, 106(4): pp. 1175-83

[80] Banerjee A, "*Can Homeopathy Bring Additional Benefit to Thalasemic Patients on Hydroxyurea Therapy? Encouraging results of a Preliminary Study,*" Evidence Based Complimentary and Alternative Medicine, October 2007

[81] www.unitedplantsavers.org

[82] Conversation with herbalist Mimi Kamp confirms many of these indications (late 1990s)

[83] Karaka B, et al, "*Enhancement of taxane-induced cytotoxicity and apoptosis by gossypol in human breast cancer line amcf-7,*" J BUON, 2009 Jul-Sep; 14(3): pp. 479-85

[84] Agnihotri VK, et al, *"Antioxidant constituents of Nymphaea caerulea flowers,"* Phytochemistry 2008 Jul; 69(10): pp 2061-6

[85] Khan N, Sultana S, *"Anticarcinogenic effect of Nymphaea alba against oxidative stress, hyperproliferative response and renal carcinogenesis in Wistar rats,"* Mol Cell Biochem 2005 Mar;271(1-2): pp.1-11

[86] Bhandarkar MR, Khan A, *"Antihepatotoxic effect of Nymphaea stellata wild., against carbon tetrachloride-induced hepatic damage in albino rats,"* J Ethnopharmacology, 2004 Mar; 91(1): pp. 61-64

[87] www.rain-tree.com

[88] Graciso Jde S, et al, *"Effects of Turnera ulmifolia L. on mouse gastric mucosa support the Turneraceae as a new source of anti-ulcerogenic drugs,"* Biol Pharm Bull, 2007 Apr, 25(4); pp. 487-91

[89] Scaglione F, Lucini V, Pannacci M, Caronno A, Leone C. *"Comparison of the potency of different brands of Serenoa repens extract on 5alpha-reductase types I and II in prostatic co-cultured epithelial and fibroblast cell,"* Pharmacology. 2008;82(4):270-5. Epub 2008 Oct 10.

[90] Abe M., et al., *"Pharmacologically relevant receptor binding characteristics and 5-alpha-reductase inhibitory activity of free fatty acids contained in saw palmetto extract,"* Biol Pham Bull 2009 Apr, 32(4); pp. 646-50

Chapter 12

[91] Schwartz Trudelle, Maureen, Molded in the Image of Changing Woman, University of Arizona Press, Tucson, 1991, p. 178

[92] Wildi E, Langer T, Schaffner W, Büter KB, *"Quantitative analysis of petasin and pyrrolizidine alkaloids in leaves and rhizomes of in situ grown Petasites hybridus plants,"* Planta Med. 1998 Apr;64(3):264-7.

[93] Debrunner, et. al., *"Sesquiterpenes of Petasites hybridus (L.) G.M. et Sch.: distribution of sesquiterpenes over plant organs,"* Pharmaceutical Acta Helvetiae, 1995, 70, pp. 167- 173

[94] No author listed, *"Monograph: Petasites hybridus (Butterbur),"* Alternative Medicine Review, 2001, Vol. 6, # 2

[95] Schapowal, Andreas, *"Randomized controlled trial of butterbur and citirzine for treating seasonal allergic rhinitis,"* BMJ, 2002 Jan 19: 324:124

[96] Anderson N, Meier T, Borlak J. , "*Toxicogenomics applied to cultures of human hepatocytes enabled an identification of novel petasites hybridus extracts for the treatment of migraine with improved hepatobiliary safety,*" Toxicol. Sci., 2009 Dec; 112(2): pp 507-20

[97] Armanni, D., et al., "*Treatment of polycystic ovary syndrome with spironolactone and licorice,*" Eur J Obstet Gynecol Reprod Biol; 2007 Mar;131(1): 61-7

Chapter 14

[98] Li, Kadota et. al., "*Effects of Cimicifuga rhizome on serum calcium and phosphate in low calcium dietary rats and on bone density in ovariectomized rats,*" Phytomedicine, 1996/97 3;4, pp. 379-385

[99] Jain NK, Singhai AK, "*Protective role of Beta vulgaris L. leaves extract and fractions on ethanol-mediated hepatic toxicity*" Acta Pol Pharm. 2012 Sep-Oct;69(5):945-50.

Chapter 15

[100] Kharrazian, Datis DHSc, DC, MS, Why Do I Still Have Thyroid Symptoms? Morgan James Publishing; Garden City, NY: 2010

[101] Panda S, Kar A, "*Changes in thyroid hormone concentrations after administration of ashwagandha root extract to adult male mice,*" J Pharm Pharmacol.,1998 Sep;50(9):1065-8.

[102] Fushiki S, "*Radiation hazards in children - Lessons from Chernobyl, Three Mile Island and Fukushima,*" Brain Dev. 2012 Oct 9. pii: S0387-7604 (12)00226-4. doi: 10.1016/j.braindev.2012.09.004. [Epub ahead of print]

[103] Cannizzaro MA, Veroux M, Costanzo M, Buffone A, Okatyeva V, "*Radiation exposure and thyroid cancer,*" Ann Ital Chir., 2012 Sep-Oct; 83(5):369-72. [Article in Italian]

Chapter 16

[104] Taylor, Leslie, Herbal Secrets of the Rain Forest, Prima Health, 1998

[105] da Silva AL, Piato AL, Bardini S, Netto CA, Nunes DS, Elisabetsky E, "*Memory retrieval improvement by Ptychopetalum olacoides in young and aging mice.*" J Ethnopharmacol. 2004 Dec;95(2-3):199-203

[106] Piato AL, Rizon LP, Martins BS, Nunes DS, Elisabetsky E, *"Antidepressant profile of Ptychopetalum olacoides Bentham (Marapuama) in mice,"* Phytother Res. 2009 Apr;23(4):519-24.

[107] Wayneberg, J., *"Contributions to the Clinical Validation of the Traditional Use of Ptychopetalum guyanna,"* Presented at the First International Congress on Ethnopharmacology, Strasbourg, France, June 5-9, 1990

[108] Manabe H, Sakagami H, Ishizone H, Kusano H, Fujimaki M, Wada C, Komatsu N, Nakashima H, Murakami T, Yamamoto N. *"Effects of Catuaba extracts on microbial and HIV infection."* In Vivo. 1992 Mar-Apr;6(2):161-5

[109] Estrada-Reyes R, Ortiz-López P, Gutiérrez-Ortíz J, Martínez-Mota L, *"Turnera diffusa Wild (Turneraceae) recovers sexual behavior in sexually exhausted males,"* J Ethnopharmacol. 2009 Jun 25;123(3):423-9

[110] Yi Y, Cao Z, Yang D, Cao Y, Wu Y, Zhao S., *"Studies on the chemical constituents of Smilax glabra,"* Yao Xue Xue Bao.1998 Nov;33(11):873-5. [Article in Chinese]

[111] Yuk SS, Lim EM, Lee JY, Lee YJ, Kim YS, Lee TH, Park SK, Bae H, Kim HM, Ko SG, Oh MS, Park W, *"Antiinflammatory effects of Epimedium brevicornum water extract on lipopolysaccharide-activated RAW264.7 macrophages,"* Phytother Res. 2010 Dec;24(12):1781-7. doi: 10.1002/ptr.3161

[112] Shu De, Ten Lectures on the Use of Medicinals from the Personal Experience of Jiao Shu De, ed. Wiseman, Nigel, & Ellis, Andrew, trans. Mitchell, Craig et al., (Taos, NM: Paradigm Publicaions 2003), p.148-9.

[113] Yin LL, Lin LL, Zhang L, Li L., *"Epimedium flavonoids ameliorate experimental autoimmune encephalomyelitis in rats by modulating neuro-inflammatory and neurotrophic responses,"* Neuropharmacology 2012 Oct;63(5):851-62. Epub 2012 Jun 21.

[114] Liu B, Zhang H, Xu C, Yang G, Tao J, Huang J, Wu J, Duan X, Cao Y, Dong J, *"Neuroprotective effects of icariin on corticosterone-induced apoptosis in primary cultured rat hippocampal neurons,"* Brain Res. 2010 Dec 20.

[115] Zhang X, Oh M, Kim S, Kim J, Kim H, Kim S, Houghton PJ, Whang W, *"Epimediphine, a novel alkaloid from Epimedium koreanum inhibits acetyl-cholinesterase,"* Nat Prod Res. 2012 Jul 24. [Epub ahead of print]

[116] Li F, Gong QH, Wu Q, Lu YF, Shi JS., "*Icariin isolated from Epimedium brevicornum Maxim attenuates learning and memory deficits induced by d-galactose in rats,*" Pharmacol Biochem Behav. 2010 Sep;96(3):301-5.

Chapter 18

[117] Edwards JE, Brown PN, Talent N, Dickinson TA, Shipley PR, "*A review of the chemistry of the genus Crataegus,*" Phytochemistry, 2012 Jul;79:5-26. doi: 10.1016/j.phytochem.2012.04.006. Epub 2012 May 18.

[118] Ibid.

Chapter 19

[119] Ou JM, Zhang XP, Wu CJ, Wu DJ, Yan P., "*Effects of dexamethasone and Salvia miltiorrhiza on multiple organs in rats with severe acute pancreatitis,*" J Zhejiang Univ Sci B. 2012 Nov;13(11):919-31. doi: 10.1631/jzus.B1100351.

[120] Proefrock, Ken N.D., "*Effective Management of the Hypertensive Patient with Botanical Medicine,*" Proceedings Manual from the Southwest Conference on Botanical Medicine, 20004, www.botanicalmedicine.org, pp. 57 - 62.

[121] Ibid.

[122] Fujita, et al, "*LKPNM: a prodrug-type ACE-inhibitory peptide derived from fish protein.,*" Immunopharmacology, 1999 Oct 15;44(1-2):123-7.

Chapter 20

[123] Youdin, K.A., et al . "*Essential fatty acids and the brain: possible health implications.,*" Int. J. Neurosci. 18: 383-399, 2000.

[124] Salem, N. Jr., et al . "*Mechanism of action of docosahexaenoic acid in the nervous system.,*" Lipids. 36(9):945-959, 2001.

[125] Reger MA, Henderson ST, Hale C, Cholerton B, Baker LD, Watson GS, Hyde K, Chapman D, Craft S, "*Effects of beta-hydroxybutyrate on cognition in memory-impaired adults,*" Neurobiol Aging. 2004 Mar;25(3):311-4.

[126] Newport, Mary T. M.D., "*Alzheimers Disease: What is there was a Cure? The Story of Ketones,*" Basic Health Publications Inc., BasicHealthPub.net

[127] Giacobini, E .(2003). *"Cholinergic function and Alzheimer's disease. International,"* Journal of Geriatric Psychiatry 18, S1-S5.

[128] Liu SH, Chang CD, Chen PH, Su JR, Chen CC, Chaung HC *"Docosahexaenoic acid and phosphatidylserine supplementations improve antioxidant activities and cognitive functions of the developing brain on pentylenetetrazol-induced seizure model,"* Brain Res. 2012 Apr 27;1451:19-26. Epub 2012 Mar 3.

[129] Gavrilova SI, Kalyn IaB, Kolykhalov IV, Roshchina IF, Selezneva ND. *"Acetyl-L-carnitine (carnicetine) in the treatment of early stages of Alzheimer's disease and vascular dementia,"* Zh Nevrol Psikhiatr Im S S Korsakova. 2011;111(9):16-22.

[130] Dong ZH, Zhang CY, Pu BH *"Effects of ginkgo biloba tablet in treating mild cognitive impairment,"* Zhongguo Zhong Xi Yi Jie He Za Zhi. 2012 Sep;32(9):1208-11.

[131] Kaur S, Chhabra R, Nehru B.,*"Ginkgo biloba extract attenuates hippocampal neuronal loss and cognitive dysfunction resulting from trimethyltin in mice,"* J. Phytomedicine. 2012 Nov 20. pii: S0944-7113(12)00369-8. doi: 10.1016/ j.phymed.2012.10.003.

[132] Kehr J, Yoshitake S, Ijiri S, Koch E, Nöldner M, Yoshitake T. *"Ginkgo biloba leaf extract (EGb 761®) and its specific acylated flavonol constituents increase dopamine and acetylcholine levels in the rat medial prefrontal cortex: possible implications for the cognitive enhancing properties of EGb 761®,"* Int Psychogeriatr. 2012 Aug;24 Suppl 1:S25-34.

[133] Bönöczk P, Panczel G, Nagy Z *"Vinpocetine increases cerebral blood flow and oxygenation in stroke patients: a near infrared spectroscopy and transcranial Doppler study,"* Eur J Ultrasound. 2002 Jun;15(1-2):85-91.

[134] Khanavi, et al., *"Cytotoxicity of Vinca minor,"* Pharm Biol, Jan 2010, Vol. 48, #1, pp. 96 - 100.

[135] Végh S, Szikszay E, Bönöczk P, Cserjés Z, Kiss G., *"Retrospective analysis of the effect of vinpocetine infusion in ophthalmologic disorders,"* Orv Hetil. 2006 Dec 10;147(49):2361-5.

[136] Song J, Xu H, Lu Q, Xu Z, Bian D, Xia Y, Wei Z, Gong Z, Dai Y *"Madecassoside suppresses migration of fibroblasts from keloids: involvement of p38 kinase and PI3K signaling pathways,"* Burns, 2012 Aug;38(5): 677-84. Epub 2012 Feb 22.

[137] Yance, Donald, Herbal Medicine, Healing, and Cancer, (Chicago: Keats, 1999), p. 131

[138] Brinker, Francis, Larrea tridentate, (Eclectic Dispensatory of Botanical Therapeutics), p. 6-141

[139] Ibid., p.6-141

[140] Van Slambrouck. S, et al, *"Effects of Crude Aqueous Medicinal Plant Extracts on Growth and Invasion of Breast Cancer Cells"*, Oncol Rep, 2007 Jun; 17(6): 1487-92

[141] Lambert JD, et al, *"Nordihydroguarietic Acid: Hepatotoxicity and Detoxification in the Mouse,"* Toxicon, 2002 Dec; 40(12) 1701-8

[142] Sheikh NM, Philen RM, Love LA, *"Chaparral Associated Hepatotoxicity,"* Arch Intern Med, 1997April 28; 157(8): 913-9

[143] Heron S, Yarnell E, *"The Safety of Low Dose Larrea tridentate (DC) Coville (creosote bush, chaparral); a Retrospective Clinical Study,"* J Altern Compliment Med, 2001 April; 7(2): 175-85

[144] Mazzio EA, Soliman KF *"In vitro screening for the tumoricidal properties of international medicinal herbs,"* Phytother Res. 2009 Mar;23(3):385-98.

[145] De Marino S, Gala F, Zollo F, Vitalini S, Fico G, Visioli F, Iorizzi M., *"Identification of minor secondary metabolites from the latex of Croton lechleri (Muell-Arg) and evaluation of their antioxidant activity,"* Molecules. 2008 Jun 1;13(6):1219-29.

[146] Wade Boyle, N.D., *"Juniper berries"* Medical Herbalism, 4(4):1,10 http://medherb.com/Materia_Medica/Juniper_Berries_-_Boyle.htm

[147] Felter, Harvey Wickes M.D., Lloyd, John.Uri Phr. M., Ph. D., King's American Dispensatory, 1898

[148] Felter, Harvey Wickes M.D., The Eclectic Materia Medica, Pharmacology and Therapeutics, 1922

[149] Cook, William, The Physiomedical Dispensatory, 1869

[150] Grieve, M., A Modern Herbal, 1931; rpt. New York: Dover, 1971

[151] Bone, Kerry, "*Juniper Berry is not a kidney irritant,*" Medial Herbalism, 07-31-94 6(2): 12 http://medherb.com/Materia_Medica/Juniperus_-_Are_juniper_berries_a_kidney_irritant_.htm

[152] Schilcher H, Leuschner F., "*The potential nephrotoxic effects of essential juniper oil.*", Arzneimittelforschung, 1997 Jul;47(7):855-8.

[153] Bone, Kerry, "*Juniper Berry is not a kidney irritant.*", Medial Herbalism, 07-31-94 6(2): 12 http://medherb.com/Materia_Medica/Juniperus_-_Are_juniper_berries_a_kidney_irritant_.htm

[154] Paul Bergner, "Juniper Berries," Medical Herbalism, 07-31-94 6(2): 13 http://medherb.com/Materia_Medica/Juniper_Berries_-_Bergner.htm

[155] Paul Bergner, "*Juniperus: Are juniper berries a kidney irritant?*", Medical Herbalism, 07-31-94 6(2): 12.

Bibliography

Allen-Hall L, Arnason JT, Cano P, Lafrenie RM., "*Uncaria tomentosa acts as a potent TNF-alpha inhibitor through NF-kappaB,*" J Ethnopharmacol. 2010 Feb 17;127 (3):685-93. Epub 2009 Dec 6.

Abe M., et al., "*Pharmacologically relevant receptor binding characteristics and 5-alpha-reductase inhibitory activity of free fatty acids contained in saw palmetto extract,*" Biol Pham Bull 2009 Apr, 32(4); pp. 646-50

Agnihotri VK, et al, "*Antioxidant constituents of Nymphaea caerulea flowers,*" Phytochemistry 2008 Jul; 69(10): pp 2061-6

Alleva, LM, Cai C, Clark IA, "*Using Complimentary and Alternative Medicines to Target Host Response during Severe Influenza,*" Evid Based Compliment Alternat Med, 2009 Sep 24

Andrews, Lynn V., Flight of the Seventh Moon, The Teachings of The Shields, Harper & Row, 1984

Antonio MA, Souza Brito AR, "*Oral anti-inflammatory and anti-ulcerogenic activities of a hydroalcoholic extract and partitioned fractions of Turnera ulmifolia (Turneraceae),*" J Ethnopharmacol, 1996 Jul, 61(3); pp. 215-28

Arletti R et al, "*Stimulating property of Turnera diffusa and Pfaffia paniculata extracts on the sexual behavior of male rats,*" Psychopharmacology (Berl), 1999 Mar, 143(1); pp. 15-9

Assilem, Melissa, Women Ripening Through Menopause, Idolatry, Inc., El Cerrito, CA, 1996

Bahorun, T., et al, "*Antioxidant Activities of Crataegus Monozyna Extracts,*" Planta Medica, 60 (1994), pp. 323-328

Bahorun, T., et al, "*Oxygen Species Scavenging activity of phenolic extracts from hawthorn fresh plant organs and pharmaceutical preparations,*" Arzneimittelforschung, 1996 Nov, 46:11, pp. 1086-9

Bernatoniene J, et al, "*The comparison of anti-oxidative kinetics in vitro of the fluid extract from maidenhair tree, motherwort and hawthorn,*" Acta Pol Pharm, 2009 Jul-Aug; 66(4): pp.415-21

Bergner, Paul, *"Influenza Prevention,"* Medical Herbalism, 2008 Summer; 15 (4)

Bernhard, H O, Thiele, K, *"Additional Flavanoids from the Leaves of Larrea tridentata,"* Planta Med, 1981 Jan; 41(1): 100-1

Bhandarkar MR, Khan A, *"Antihepatotoxic effect of Nymphaea stellata wild., against carbon tetrachloride-induced hepatic damage in albino rats,"* J Ethnopharmacology, 2004 Mar; 91(1): pp. 61-64

Boericke, William, M.D., Materia Medica with Repertory, Santa Rosa, California, Boericke and Tafel, Inc., 1927

Bone, Kerry, Clinical Applications of Ayurvedic & Chinese Herbs, Monographs for the Western Practitioner, Warwick, Queensland, Australia, Phytotherapy Press, 1996

Bonheim, Jalaja, Aphrodite's Daughters, Simon & Schuster, 1997

Brinker, Francis, N.D., Larrea Tridentata, Creosote Bush, monograph, Eclectic Dispensatory of Therapeutics, Sandy, Oregon

Bystritsky A, Kerwin L, Feusner JD, *"A pilot study of Rhodiola rosea (Rhodax) for generalized anxiety disorder (GAD),"* Journal of Alternative and Complimentary Medicine, March 2006: 14(2); pp. 175-80

Camacho-Corona, M del R, et al, *"Activity Against Drug-Resistant Tuberculosis Strain of Plants Used in Mexican Traditional Medicine to Treat Tuberculosis and Other Respiratory Diseases"*, Phytother Res, 2008 Jan; 22(1): 82-5

Chernen, Kim, The Hungry Self, Women Eating and Identity, Harper & Row, 1985

Clarke, John Henry, M.D., A Dictionary of Practical Materia Medica, Vol. I, New Delhi: Indian Books and Periodicals Syndicate

Crawford, Amanda McQuade, M.N.I.M.H., Herbal Remedies for Women, Prima Health, Rocklin, CA 1997

Dallett, Janet O., When The Spirits Come Back, Inner City Books, Toronto, 1988

Delwiche, C.C., Zinke, P.J., Johnson, C.M., "*Nitrogen fixation by Ceanothus,*" Plant Physiol., Nov. 1964; 40 (6): pp. 1045 - 1047.

Diamant, Anita, The Red Tent, Picador, USA, NY, 1997

Estrada-Reyes R, et al, "*Turnera diffusa Wild (Turneraceae) recovers sexual behavior in sexually exhausted males,*" (rat study), J Ethnopharm, 2009Jun 25, 123(3); pp. 423-9

Felter HW, MD, The Eclectic Materia Medica, Pharmacology, and Therapeutics, Eclectic Medical Publications 1985

Flinders, Carol Ann, At The Root of This Longing, Reconciling a Spiritual Hunger and a Feminist Thirst, Harper Collins, San Francisco, 1998

Gabor, M., "*Pharmacologic Effects of Flavanoids on Blood Vessels,*" Symposia Angiologica Santoriana, 4th Int. Symp., Fribourg - Nyon 1972, Angiologica 9: 355-374 (223-242) 1972

Gladstar, Rosemary, Herbal Healing for Women, Simon & Schuster, N.Y., 1993

Graciso Jde S, et al, "*Effects of Turnera ulmifolia L. on mouse gasttic mucosa support the Turneraceae as a new source of anti-ulcerogenic drugs,*" Biol Pharm Bull, 2007 Apr, 25(4); pp. 487-91

Grieve, M., A Modern Herbal , Vol. I & II. 2 vols. 1931; rpt. New York: Dover , 1971.

Green, James, The Male Herbal, Crossing Press, Freedom, CA, 1991

Griffin, Susan, Woman and Nature: The Roaring Inside Her, Women's Press, London, 1984

Heron, S, Yarnell, E, "*The Safety of Low Dose Larrea tridentata (DC) Coville (Creosote Bush or Chaparral): a Retrospective Clinical Study*", J Altern Compliment Med, 2001 April; 7(2): 175-85

Hobbs, Christopher, L.Ac., Goldberg, Alicia, Mcguffin, Michael, Upton, Roy, Botanical Safety Handbook, American Herbal Products Association, CRC Press LLC., Boca Taton, Fla, 1997

Hobbs, Christopher, L.Ac., Medicinal Mushrooms, An Exploration of Tradition, Healing, and Culture, Interweave Press, Inc., Loveland, Colorado, 1986

Hoffman, David, An Elder's Herbal, Healing Arts Press, Rochester, VT 1993

Jung, Carl Gustaf, Memories, Dreams and Reflections, Vintage Books, New York, 1965

Mendell, Arnold, Working With The Dreaming Body, London, Penguin Books, 1985

Kenner, Dan and Requena, Yves, Botanical Medicine, A European Professional Perspective, Paradigm Publications, Brookline, MA, 1996

Kinstler, Clysta, The Moon Under Her Feet, Harper, San Francisco, 1983

Kohanov, Linda, The Tao of Equus, New World World Library, Novato, CA, 2001

Kuhnau, Joachim, *"The Flavanoids: A Class of Semi-Essential Food Components: Their Role in Human Nutrition"*, Wld Rev. Nutr. Diet, vol. 24, pp. 117-191 (1976)

Lad, Dr. Vasant, and Frawley, David, The Yoga of Herbs, Lotus Press, Santa Fe, 1986

Karaka B, et al, *"Enhancement of taxane-induced cytotoxicity and apoptosis by gossypol in human breast cancer line amcf-7,"* J BUON, 2009 Jul-Sep; 14(3): pp. 479-85

Khan N, Sultana S, *"Anticarcinogenic effect of Nymphaea alba against oxidative stress, hyperproliferative response and renal carcinogenesis in Wistar rats,"* Mol Cell Biochem 2005 Mar;271(1-2): pp.1-11

Laferriere JE, Weber CW, Kohlhepp EA, *"Mineral composition of some traditional Mexican teas,"* Plant Foods Hum Nutr, 1991 Jul; 41(3): pp. 277-82

Lambert, J D, et al, *"Nordihydroguairetic Acid: Hepatotoxicity and Detoxification in the Mouse"*, Toxican, 2002 Dec; 40(12): 1701-1708

Lindlahr, Henry M.D., Philosophy of Natural Therapies, Maidstone Osteopathic Clinic Publisher, Maidstone, Kent, 1975, p. 121

Li JX, et. al., *"Triterpenoids from Cimicifuga rhizome, a novel class of inhibitors on bone resorption and ovariectomized bone loss,"* Maturitas; 2007 Sep 20, 58 (1), pp. 59 - 69

Li XC, Cai L, Wu CD, "*Antimicrobial compounds from C. americanus against oral pathogens,*" Phytochemistry, 1997, Sep.; 46(1): pp. 97-102.

Lookingbill Donald P., M.D., & Marks, James G., M.D. Principles of Dermatology, W.B.Saunders Company, Philadelphia, 1986

Lust, J., The Herb Book, 1974; rpt. New York: Bantam, 1979.

Lynch, TA, Miya TS, Carr CJ, "*An investigation of the blood coagulating principles from C. americanus,*" J. Amer. Pharm. Assoc., Amer. Pharm. Assoc., Baltimore.

Mao QQ, et al, "*Peony glycosides produce anti-depressant-like action in mice exposed to chronic unpredictable mild stress: effects on hypothalamic-pituitary-adrenal function and brain-derived neurotrophic factor,*" Prog Neuropsychopharmacol Biol Psychiatry, 2009 Oct 1, 33(7); pp. 1211-6

McQuade-Crawford, Amanda, MNIMH, Herbal Remedies for Women, Prima, Rocklin, CA, 1997

Middleton, Elliott Jr., "*The Flavanoids,*" Trends in Pharmacologic Sciences, August 1984, pp. 335-338

Mitchell, William A., N.D., Plant Medicine in Practice, Using the Teachings of John Bastyr, Churchill Livingstone, Philadelphia, 1993

Monaghan, Patricia, The Book of Goddesses and Heroines, New York, E.P. Dutton, 1981

Moore, Michael, Medicinal Plants of The Pacific West, Santa Fe, Red Crane Books

Moore, Michael, Medicinal Plants of the Desert and Canyon West, Santa Fe, Museum of New Mexico Press, 1989

Nascimento MA, et al, "*Turnera ulmifolia L. (Turneraceae): preliminary study of its anti-oxidant activity,*" Bioresour Technol, 2006 Aug, 97(12); pp 1387-91

Noble, Vicki, Motherpeace: A Way to the Goddess Through Myth, Art and Tarot, Harper and Row, San Francisco, 1985

Oktyabrsky O., et al, "*Assessment of anti-oxidant activity of plants using microbial test systems,*" J Applied Microbiol, 2009 Apr, 106(4): pp. 1175-83
Owen, Lara, Honoring Menstruation, Harper Collins, San Francisco, 1993

Panossian A, Wikman G, Sarris J., "*Rosenroot (Rhodiola rosea): traditional use, chemical compoeition, pharmacology, and clinical efficacy,*" Phytomedicine, June 2010: 17(7); pp. 241-93

Patai, Raphael, The Hebrew Goddess, Wayne State University Press, Detroit, 1967

Philip, Hazel, N.D., L.Ac., "*Hot Flashes: A Review of the Literature on Alternative and Complimentary Treatment Approaches*", Alternative Medicine Review, Vol. 8, No. 3, August 2003, p. 284

Piacente S, et al, "*Flavanoids and arbutin from Turnera diffusa,*" Z Naturforsch C, 2002 Nov - Dec, 57(11-12); pp. 963-5

Pizzorno & Murray, Encyclopedia of Natural Medicine, Prima Publishing, 1998

Qiu SX, et al, "*A triterpene glycoside from black cohosh that inhibits osteoclastoegensis by modulating RANKL and TNF alfa-signaling pathways,*" Chem Biol, 2007 Jul 14(7), pp. 860-9

Ritter M et al, "*Cardiac and Electrophysiological Effects of Primary and Refined Extracts from Leonurus cardiac L. (Ph.Eur.),*" Planta Med, 2009 Nov 16

Roschek B Jr, Fink RC, McMichael MD, Li D, Alberte RS, "*Elderberry flavonoids bind to and prevent H1N1 infection in vitro,*" Phytochemistry, 2009 Jul;70(10):1255-61. Epub 2009 Aug 12.

Schaef, Anne Wilson, Women's Reality, An Emerging Female System in a White Male Society, Harper, San Francisco, 1981, 1985, 1992

Sheikh, N M, Philen, R M, Love, L A, "*Chaparral Associated Hepatotoxicity,*" Arch Intern Med, 1997 April; 157(8): 913-9

Sherman, John, N.D., The Complete Botanical Prescriber, 3rd ed., Sherman 1993

Smith, Ed, Therapeutic Herb Manual, Ed Smith, Williams Oregon, 1999
Stengler, Mark, The Health Benefits of Medicinal Mushrooms, Basic Health Publications, Inc., North Bergen, N.J., 2005

Schwarz, Maureen Trudelle, Molded in the Image of Changing Woman: Navajo Views on the Human Body and Personhood, University of Arizona Press, Tucson, 1997

Shlain, Leonard, The Alphabet Versus The Goddess, N.Y., 1998

Taylor, Leslie, Herbal Secrets of the Rainforest, Prima Publishing, Rocklin, CA 1998

Tilgner, S., Herbal Medicine from the Heart of the Earth, Creswell, OR: Wise Acres Press, 1999.

Trickey, Ruth, Women, Hormones, and the Menstrual Cycle, Allen & Unwin, Crows Nest, NSW, Australia, 2003

Van Slambrouck S., et al, "*Effects of Crude Aqueous Medicinal Plant Extracts on Growth and Invasion of Breast Cancer Cells,*" Oncol Rep, 2007 Jun; 17 (6): 1487-92

Walker, Barbara, The Woman's Encyclopedia of Myths and Secrets

Weed, Susun, Menopausal Years, The Wise Woman Way, Ash Tree Publishing, Woodstock, N.Y., 1992

Whitmont, Edward C., Return of the Goddess, Crossroad, NY, 1984

Wood, Matthew, The Book of Herbal Wisdom, Using Plants as Medicine, North Atlantic Books, Berkeley, 1997

Wren, R.C., F.L.S., revised by Williamson, Elizabeth M. B.Sc., Ph.D., et al, Potter's New Cyclopaedia of Botanical Drugs and Preparations, Essex, England, C.W. Daniel Company Ltd., 1989

Wuttke, W., Seidlova-Wuttke, D., Gorkow, C., "*The Cimicifuga preparation BNO 1055 vs. conjugated estrogens in a double blind placebo controlled study: effects on menopause symtoms and bone markers,*" Maturitas, 2003 Mar 14; 44 Suppl 1: pp. 567-77

Yance, Donald, Jr., C.N., M.H., A.H.G., with Valentine, Arlene, Herbal Medicine, Healing, and Cancer, A Comprehensive Program for Prevention and Treatment, Chicago, Keats Publishing, 1999

Zhao J, et al, "*Anti-aromatase activity of the constituents from damiana (Turnera diffusa)*," J Ethnopharm, 2008 Dec 8, 120(3); pp. 387 - 93

Zhao J, et al, "*Phytochemical investigation of Turnera diffusa*," J Nat Prod, 2007 Feb, 70(2); pp. 289-92

GENERAL INDEX

C

PLANT INDEX

Common Names

Latin Names

Plant Families

INDEX of HOMEOPATHIC REMEDIES

73711345R00168

Made in the USA
Columbia, SC
17 July 2017